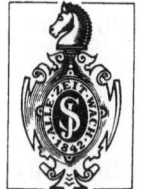

Clinical Practice in Urology
Series Editor: Geoffrey D. Chisholm

Current Perspectives in Paediatric Urology

Edited by
Robert H. Whitaker

With 36 Figures

Springer-Verlag
London Berlin Heidelberg New York
Paris Tokyo Hong Kong

Robert H. Whitaker, MD, MChir, FRCS
Consultant Paediatric Urologist, Department of Urology,
Addenbrooke's Hospital, Hills Road, Cambridge CB2 2QQ

Series Editor
Geoffrey D. Chisholm, ChM, FRCS, FRCS Ed
Professor of Surgery, University of Edinburgh; and Consultant
Urological Surgeon, Western General Hospital,
Edinburgh, Scotland

Cover: Fig. 5.2b. IVU of a child to show a right-sided hydronephrosis due to obstruction of the pelvi-ureteric junction.

British Library Cataloguing in Publication Data
Current perspectives in paediatric urology.
1. Paediatrics. Urology
I. Whitaker, Robert H.
618.92'6

Library of Congress Cataloging-in-Publication Data
Current perspectives in paediatric urology/Robert H. Whitaker (ed.).
p.   cm. — (Clinical practice in urology).   Includes bibliographies and index.

ISBN-13: 978-1-4471-1714-8   e-ISBN-13: 978-1-4471-1712-4
DOI: 10.1007/978-1-4471-1712-4

1. Pediatric urology. I. Whitaker, R. H. (Robert H.) II. Series. [DNLM:
1. Urologic Diseases—in infancy & childhood.   WS 320   C976]   RJ466.C87   1989
618.92'6—dc20
DNLM/DLC
for Library of Congress   89-19692
                                                                            CIP

Springer-Verlag London Ltd, Springer House, 8 Alexandra Road,
London SW19 7JZ, UK.

© Springer-Verlag Berlin Heidelberg 1989
Softcover reprint of the hardcover 1st edition 1989

Filmset by MJS Publications, Buntingford, Herts., UK
Printed by Biddles Ltd, Guildford, Surrey, UK

2128/3916-543210   Printed on acid-free paper

Series Editor's Foreword

The aim of this series is to bring the reader up-to-date data and opinions on the practice of urological surgery. The ten titles published since 1982 have all been concerned with adult urology, with reference to paediatric problems included in some relevant chapters. The addition of this title on paediatric urology is especially welcome because it brings together the important components of the sub-specialty.

This book has developed from one of the first of the annual courses in urological sub-specialties provided for trainees in the UK as part of their higher surgical training. But that audience is not the only one at which this book is aimed. In his Preface, Robert Whitaker emphasises the changes over the past ten to fifteen years: this means that any urologist over the age of 45 is already out of date in much of his or her knowledge of paediatric urology – unless there has been a genuine attempt at continuing medical education. Attendance and discussions at meetings and reading of current literature are useful methods of updating our knowledge. However, this book provides a much-needed link with the paediatric urology course and is a splendid reference source for all urologists.

Robert Whitaker has gathered together four eminent co-authors to present their material on the main issues in paediatric urology. In keeping with the aims of this series, the data are up to date, the perspectives are contemporary and in every way this is an excellent addition to Clinical Practice in Urology.

Edinburgh, 1989   Geoffrey D. Chisholm

Preface

Many aspects of urology are advancing so fast that standard textbooks are often lamentably out-of-date by the time they are published. This is particularly true in paediatric urology, where prenatal diagnosis has altered our whole approach to several conditions. There have been advances in the management of hypospadias and Wilms' Tumour that would make their management unrecognisable to those practising 15 years ago. This rapid progress has led to a profusion of shorter texts that examine the advances in a few topics at a time, often in depth.

This book is based on an annual two-day paediatric urology course, now in its fifth year, organised in Great Britain for senior registrars in urology and paediatric surgery and for consultants who choose, or are obliged, to deal with urological problems in children.

The topics chosen are those that are either most controversial, for example, prenatal diagnosis and the management of neonatal hydronephrosis, or historically difficult to understand, such as intersex. The course has been popular and well-attended and its success has been in no small part due to the enthusiasm of the speakers, who are responsible for busy paediatric urological practices and try to keep in the forefront of advances in the subject. The course has now been taken under the wing of the Standing Committee on Postgraduate Education and the British Association of Urological Surgeons as one of its five major teaching commitments.

We are pleased that the text from this course has been included in the Clinical Practice in Urology Series and trust that it will complement the other excellent texts published in it.

Cambridge, 1989   Robert H. Whitaker

Contents

Contributors

David C. S. Gough, FRCS, FRCS(E), FRACS, DCH
Consultant Paediatric Surgeon, Royal Manchester Children's
Hospital, Pendlebury, Manchester M27 1HA

Philip G. Ransley, FRCS
Consultant Paediatric Urologist, The Hospital for Sick Children,
Great Ormond Street, London WC1

David F. M. Thomas, MRCP, FRCS
Consultant Paediatric Urologist/Surgeon, St. James's University
Hospital, Beckett Street, Leeds LS9 7TF

Robert H. Whitaker, MD, MChir, FRCS
Consultant Paediatric Urologist, Department of Urology,
Addenbrooke's Hospital, Hills Road, Cambridge CB2 2QQ

Chapter 1

Reflux and Duplex Systems

David F. M. Thomas and Robert H. Whitaker

Duplications

General Principles

Duplication of the upper urinary tract can be divided into complete and incomplete. The embryology of the defects is complex and is not within the scope of this chapter. Duplications arise from a fault in the ureteric bud with the bifid ureteric bud giving rise to a duplex system; the level at which the ureteric bud divides into two determines whether it is a complete or incomplete duplication. Duplications are common and occur in 1 in 125 (0.8%) live births. In the vast majority of patients they are asymptomatic and require no surgical intervention. It is important to note that the upper pole system drains by the most distal of the two ureters and the lower pole system drains by the shorter and more proximal one. This rule, the Meyer Weigart Law, has clinical implications (Fig. 1.1). Often the two ureters open in close proximity to each other and there are no problems associated with this. However, when complications do occur, they are quite predictable. The upper pole ureter which opens more distally is more likely to be associated with obstruction in its long sub-mucosal tunnel. Alternatively, its opening may be ectopic. Thus, it is the upper pole system that always drains via an ectopic ureter. In practice the upper pole system is frequently dysplastic particularly if associated with a ureterocele and less than 10% of these upper systems have any useful function. If, however, the upper pole ureter is draining in a relatively normal site, upper pole function is often preserved. The changes in the upper pole are not due to acquired obstruction; there is inherent dysplasia due to the fact that the abnormal

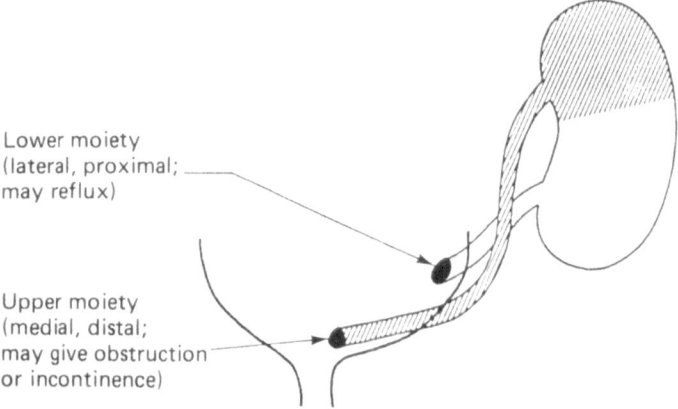

Lower moiety
(lateral, proximal;
may reflux)

Upper moiety
(medial, distal;
may give obstruction
or incontinence)

Fig. 1.1. Meyer Weigart Law.

ureteric bud has made contact with a poor bit of the developing kidney (Snyder 1985).

The lower pole system drains via the more proximal ureter and the submucosal tunnel may be shorter than normal so that reflux may occur. Reflux, thus, is predominantly the complication of the lower pole. It is, however, possible on occasion to have reflux into both the ureters.

The incidence of *ureterocele* is shown in Table 1.1. It is six times more commonly unilateral than bilateral and is equally common on each side. It is more frequently seen in females than in males. Most ureteroceles are associated with a duplex system but there is an entity called the "simple" or "orthotopic ureterocele" that is not associated with a duplex system. Another condition to be differentiated from the duplex system is the *single ectopic ureter*, a rare entity in which the ectopia of the ureter is not associated with duplication of the urinary tract. The ureter in this situation may open into the bladder neck or urethra. It is a condition which is predominantly seen in females, often in association with a small bladder and a poorly formed bladder neck. Even after reimplantation of these ureters into the bladder, the girls are frequently incontinent and some form of surgery is usually needed for the bladder neck.

Table 1.1. Ureterocele

Incidence	1:4000
Female:male	4:1
Duplex	70%
Simple	20%–40%
Ectopic	60%–80%

Fig. 1.2 shows the classical intravenous urogram (IVU) appearances of a duplex system. When there is duplication on one side, duplication on the opposite side should be suspected. An IVU shows the typical appearances of a ureterocele in the bladder and the so-called "drooping flower" appearances of the right lower pole calices. The non-functioning upper part of the kidney does not show on the X-ray film.

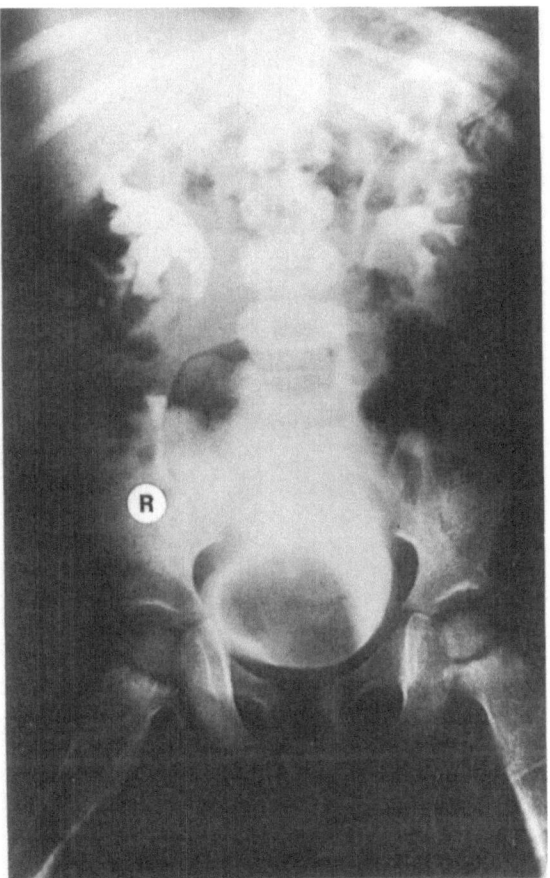

Fig. 1.2. Intravenous urogram showing duplex system on left side. On the right, calices are displaced downwards, outwards (drooping flower), the right ureter is displaced and there is a filling defect in the bladder. These are the classical signs of a right ectopic ureterocele.

Presentation

Most children with duplication present with symptoms of infection which is due to reflux into the lower pole or to obstruction and stasis in an upper pole system. Nowadays, duplications are frequently detected on a prenatal scan. However, some children may present with urinary incontinence from an ectopic ureter draining below the bladder neck. A plum-coloured introital swelling in a female may be a prolapsed ectopic ureterocele (Fig. 1.3). At first an imperforate hymen may be suspected or possibly a hydrocolpos. These are possibilities, but it is far more likely to be a prolapsed ectopic ureterocele. Although this is not a common presentation, it is important that it should be recognised.

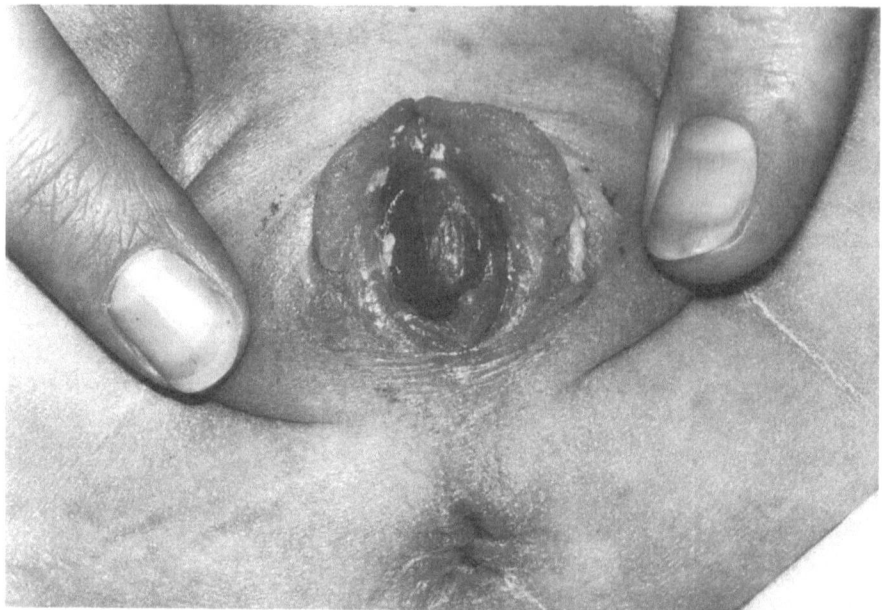

Fig. 1.3.   Prolapsed ureterocele showing at introitus.

Investigation

The investigation of these conditions is the same as for the investigation of any child with a urinary tract infection. *Ultrasound* is extremely useful for investigating duplications. The upper pole may be difficult to identify by any other modality and it certainly may not be seen on an IVU if it is non-functioning. Ultrasound also shows the dilated upper pole ureter and the ureterocele within the bladder. A *micturating cystogram* is essential to detect reflux which is such a common complication of duplication. It is usually confined to the lower pole, but occasionally it will be into both moieties of a duplex kidney. An IVU is still mandatory to give details of the anatomy of the non-dilated ureter or ureters. Furthermore, some form of functional assessment is needed, if surgery is to be contemplated, to give details of the distribution of function between the various moieties and a *DMSA (dimercaptosuccinate) scan* gives such an accurate assessment. An IVU often remains the best way of demonstrating a ureterocele; during a micturating cystogram the ureterocele may be compressed by bladder pressure and disappear. The ureterocele may obstruct the bladder neck and this may be severe enough to give upper tract dilatation or even renal failure. Dilatation of the lower pole system in the presence of a ureterocele is more commonly due to an outflow obstruction than direct obstruction of its ureter by the ureterocele itself.

Management

Ureterocele

After the diagnosis is fully substantiated a decision must be made as to the best form of surgery. There is no place for conservative management in a symptomatic child with an ectopic ureterocele. Thus, in a child with a poorly functioning upper pole associated with a ureterocele, with or without reflux into one or more of the other ureters, the decision is between a major operation involving a hemi-nephroureterectomy with excision of the ureterocele, or a simplified approach in which the upper pole system and as much ureter as possible is removed from a loin incision (Fig. 1.4). The ureterocele in this simplified operation is left intact in the hope that it will collapse down and give no further problems. The former operation, hemi-nephro-ureterectomy, is one of the largest operations in paediatric urology and involves two incisions.

During the dissection of the upper pole, it is important to stay near to the kidney and identify separately the vessels to each half of the kidney. It is useful to divide the ectopic ureter early and manipulate it to expose the upper pole. A line of demarcation is usually obvious between the upper and lower poles. The upper pole renal capsule is incised and the abnormal upper pole tissue removed down to the junction with the lower pole. If a lower pole calix is accidentally opened at this stage, it can easily be closed with continuous chromic catgut. Haemostasis is secured using under-running sutures or bi-polar diathermy. Mattress chromic catgut sutures are used to approximate the edges of the lower pole. The ureter is then dissected down as far as possible. If the major procedure is to be carried out then the loin incision is closed at this stage and a second incision in the lower abdomen is made to gain access to the bladder and the ureterocele which needs to be excised. Intra- and extra-vesical dissection is needed so that the blood supply of the lower pole ureter is safeguarded. The dissection should stay extremely close to the ectopic ureter. The lower pole ureter nearly always needs reimplanting after excision of the ureterocele and closure of the defect in the bladder wall. Reflux is likely to be induced by the dissection even if it were not present before. A Cohen reimplant is a satisfactory procedure in this situation. The detrusor muscle at the site of entry of the ectopic ureter needs to be carefully reconstructed before the mucosa is closed over it.

The disadvantages of the major procedure are that the lower pole ureter may be jeopardised and, with a low dissection, continence may be compromised, particularly if the ectopic ureter is running down through the bladder neck and striated sphincter mechanism. In some girls the ureter runs down between the urethra and the vagina presenting an extremely difficult dissection. In this situation continence can easily be compromised. Because of these potential complications it has become popular, particularly in the USA, to opt for a more simple operation of upper pole partial nephrectomy and excision of the upper ureter leaving the distal ureter and the ureterocele intact (Fig. 1.4). It is assumed that once the ureterocele collapses it will not interfere with voiding. This simple approach is attractive but is not without its problems.

Clearly coincidental reflux is not being treated. Thus, there is a 25%–50% re-operation rate mostly to correct the reflux but occasionally for complications in association with the remaining upper pole ureter and ureterocele. Some

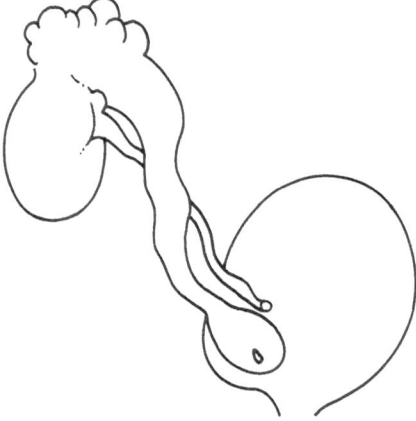

Heminephrectomy only
(simplified approach)

Heminephroureterectomy
(ureterocele excised, lower
pole ureter reimplanted)

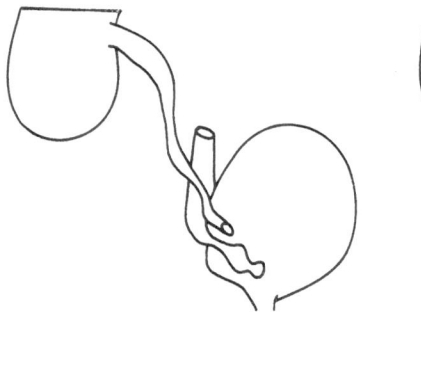

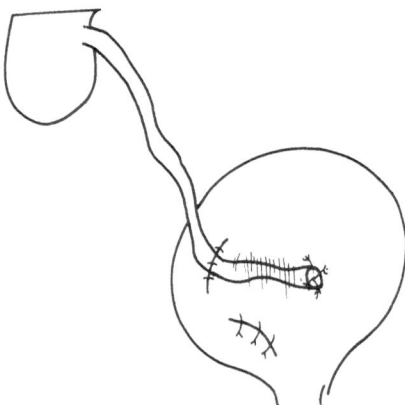

50% Lower pole reflux
25%-50% need secondary operation

Major procedure
Risk of incontinence
Risk of damage to lower pole ureter

Fig. 1.4. Management options for ectopic ureterocele.

guidelines for the selection of operation type are needed. In a small ureterocele with a relatively non-dilated ureter, the simple approach is probably satisfactory. In the presence of a large ureterocele or gross reflux, the full operation is probably more appropriate.

Duplex without Ureterocele

In an ectopic system in the absence of a ureterocele, a simple upper pole partial nephrectomy is all that is needed with excision of the ureter as far as reasonable through a loin incision. The lower part of a refluxing ectopic ureter should probably be excised but extensive dissection should be avoided because of the risk of damaging sphincter or ejaculatory mechanisms. A small stump of 2–3 cm of ectopic ureter can safely be left.

Reflux into the lower pole of a duplex system can be managed conservatively but there is probably less chance of spontaneous cessation into such a ureter than there is with a simple system. If a reimplant is to be performed, it is essential to reimplant both ipsi-lateral ureters together since they are in a common sheath (Fig. 1.5). An attempt to separate these ureters would jeopardise the blood supply of each ureter. The operation is only a little more difficult than reimplanting a single ureter. The ureters are dissected as for a Cohen reimplantation. The alternative is to remove the lower pole of the kidney and this is where a DMSA scan is particularly useful for assessing the amount of functioning tissue. If it is non-functioning or poorly functioning it may be more appropriate to perform a lower pole partial nephrectomy. The ureter will, of course, need to be removed down to the bladder. A lower pole partial nephrectomy alone would not be appropriate in this situation as it would leave a long refluxing stump of ureter. On rare occasions it might be appropriate to perform a pyelo-pyelostomy with excision of the refluxing ureter as low as possible. Anastomosis of the refluxing ureter to the non-refluxing ureter low in the pelvis is probably not a satisfactory procedure as it may jeopardise the well-functioning upper pole.

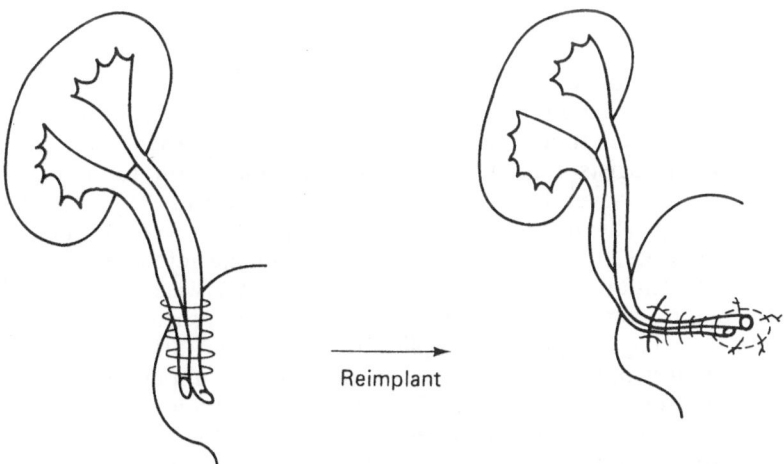

Reimplant

Fig. 1.5. Reflux into lower pole ureter. Treatment options are conservative or operative (re-implantation of both ureters, hemi-nephro-ureterectomy or pyelopyelostomy). The most commonly performed operation is a double-barrelled reimplantation, illustrated in this figure.

Finally, if there are unusual IVU appearances, or the presentation seems unusual, the possibility of a duplex system should always be considered.

The *methylene blue test* is sometimes appropriate in paediatric urology. A Foley catheter is placed in the bladder and some saline mixed with methylene blue is instilled into the bladder. A pad is then placed on the perineum. If, after half an hour, the pad is damp but has clear urine upon it, it can be inferred that this urine has come from an ectopic ureter. It should be noted that an ectopic ureter is a rare cause of incontinence, even in girls. There will be certain clues in the history. For instance, these girls have never had a dry day in their lives. The incontinence may be worse by day than at night and, of course, they can void normally but be continuously wet between times. It should be possible to make the diagnosis from investigation by IVU alone or together with an ultrasound, but if there is doubt then the methylene blue test can be performed.

The most common drainage sites for ectopic ureters differ according to the sex of the patient. In boys, an ectopic ureter is less common but it can drain into the region of the prostatic urethra, the vas or seminal vesicle so that the boy may present with epididymo-orchitis but not incontinence. In girls, incontinence can occur if the ureter drains below the bladder neck and particularly if it is below the main sphincter mechanisms. The ureter may also, of course, drain directly into the vagina or at the introitus. Occasionally, in girls it is possible to demonstrate the site of the opening and pass a fine catheter into it. Some ectopic ureters in girls pass down between the vagina and the urethra and the dissection of such a low ureter is both hazardous and inadvisable. However, on occasions it is necessary to remove it, in which case the trans-trigonal approach with splitting of the trigone is most appropriate. In boys, an ectopic ureter sometimes ends in a cystic mass behind the bladder involving the seminal vesicle. This mass should not be removed for fear of interfering with the ejaculatory mechanisms. In boys, there may be a spurious incontinence in the presence of an ectopic ureter opening into the posterior urethra. It may lead to a reflex contraction of the bladder giving the impression of incontinence.

A staged procedure for the more major operation for ectopic ureterocele may be appropriate: for example, occasionally, with a severely infected system, the upper pole of the kidney may be removed as a first procedure and the lower ureter at a later time. Some of these children do present with gross sepsis and some urologists regard this as the only indication for doing a staged procedure. In a severely ill, infected child, it is possible to uncap the ureterocele endoscopically to allow the pus to escape. However, nowadays, with modern antibiotics, it is usually possible to overcome infection without any operative intervention. The ureterocele should not otherwise be uncapped since it immediately commits the surgeon to the major procedure and no longer makes the simple approach applicable. A further alternative is a percutaneous nephrostomy for drainage of pus in the upper tract. The problem here, however, is that not all these upper systems are hydro-nephrotic. Some are really quite small and dysplastic and the placement of a percutaneous tube would then be extremely difficult or impossible. The residual bladder mucosa at the bladder neck after excision of the ureterocele can be dealt with endoscopically with a diathermy electrode or re-sectoscope.

Reflux

It is important to appreciate that there are two sites for reflux in the urinary tract. The first is the *ureterovesical junction* and the second is within the kidney itself. The ureterovesical junction functions effectively as a flap valve. It is the intravesical pressure that compresses the intramural part of the ureter against the detrusor and this prevents reflux occurring normally. In addition, there seems to be an active component at the time of voiding. As the bladder neck opens, the trigonal fibres which are attached to the lower edge of the ureter have the effect of pulling the ureter down inside Waldeyer's sheath and effectively lengthening the intramural course of the ureter. Reflux occurs because this intramural portion is too short; in most instances this is due to an embryological defect. During the last 15 years it has become clear that we must also consider reflux from the collecting system back into the parenchyma of the kidney itself and this is the phenomenon of *intra-renal reflux*. It is due to the work of Hodson, latterly in the USA, and Philip Ransley and Tony Risdon in the UK that we know so much more about intra-renal reflux and its relationship with the morphology of the renal papilla.

The normal renal papilla in the human adult is conical shaped and the collecting ducts enter it obliquely (Fig. 1.6a). This in turn imparts an anti-reflux mechanism. However, in certain parts of the kidney in children, particularly in the poles of the kidney, it is possible to find abnormal papillae. These are flat, so-called compound papillae (Fig. 1.6b), in which the collecting ducts enter almost at right angles; this is a situation which allows reflux of infected urine right into the renal parenchyma. This may be an over-simplification of the situation as it is sometimes difficult to distinguish between the normal and this abnormal type of papilla. It is possible to demonstrate the contrast passing into the parenchyma on a micturating cystogram. But the question that needs to be asked is why this phenomenon is not observed more often: it is only seen in 5%–10% of cases of reflux on cystography. The answer probably is that sufficiently high pressures are not used and the amount of contrast entering the parenchyma is probably small compared with the total amount of contrast that is seen on the X-ray film. However, experimentally, intra-renal reflux does seem to play a crucial role in the genesis of renal scarring.

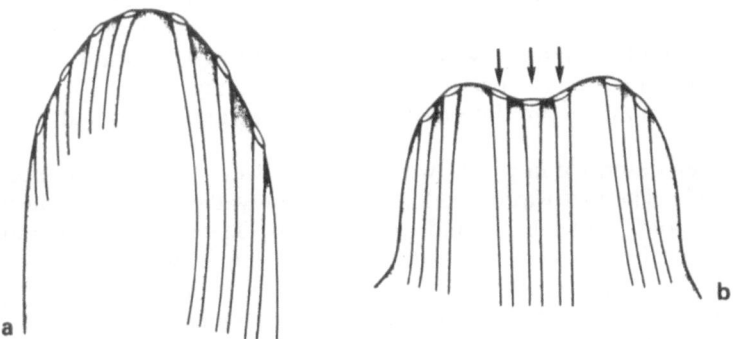

Fig. 1.6a. Normal papilla.   **b.** Abnormal (compound) papilla.

It is possible to get some idea of the *incidence of reflux* from sibling studies when siblings without symptoms have been investigated. In such siblings that have reflux, some 70% of them are asymptomatic (Jenkins and Noe 1982). Thus, reflux would appear to be more common than one would suspect from the number of children who present with urinary tract infection. In a series of children with urinary tract infections, the infection is associated with reflux in 30% (McKerrow et al. 1984). However, much depends on the age of the group of children being investigated. Thus, the younger the age group, the more likely reflux is to be found. In older children infection is much more likely to be due to some other problem, such as dysfunctional voiding, than to reflux. There is scarring at the time of presentation in 10%–15% of female children with reflux and of these 0.1% go on to develop chronic renal failure. An excellent article by Kincaid-Smith (1983) considered the epidemiology of reflux.

We have considered the anatomical factors and it now appears clear that other factors play a role in reflux (Table 1.2). Perhaps the most important of these is the *bladder behaviour*. The relationship between the lower urinary tract and the upper urinary tract is very important. In a proportion of cases it may be that the infection itself is causing the reflux rather than the result of it.

Voiding abnormalities have been investigated fully in the USA and in some studies there has been a 50% incidence of reflux in girls with such voiding disorders (Koff et al. 1979). Thus, voiding disorders and reflux go hand-in-hand in the particular age group of 3–8-year-old children.

Table 1.2. Aetiological factors in reflux

Anatomical	Short intramural ureter
Functional	Increased voiding pressures
	Instability
Infective	Bacterial adherence

There seem to be two peak incidences of reflux. There is an early peak which represents children with gross anatomical abnormalities; this group includes boys in at least equal number to girls. A second peak of incidence is later in childhood and consists almost entirely of girls, many of whom have voiding disorders. It is simple to imagine that if the vesico-ureteric junction has a slightly inadequate sub-mucosal length it only needs a little pressure within the bladder to tip it from a non-refluxing junction to a refluxing one. One type of abnormality which can precipitate reflux is detrusor sphincter dyssynergia which may or may not be combined with detrusor instability. High intra-vesical pressure may be either sustained, perhaps associated with a degree of sphincter over-activity, or it may be an intermittent high pressure associated with voiding.

A study has been described in which two cystograms were performed in each child (Hanna 1984). The first was carried out within a few days of presentation with urinary infection; 21 of the 27 children had reflux. The second cystogram was performed after the infection had settled, between 4 and 6 weeks later, and showed that 6 of the children no longer had reflux. Thus, reflux is not simply due to an anatomical abnormality but there are a number of inter-related functional factors such as abnormal voiding that may give rise to reflux. Reflux gives rise to infection which may lead to bladder irritability and that, in turn,

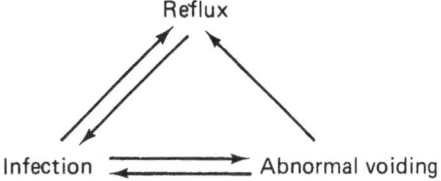

Fig. 1.7. A vicious circle of problems in reflux.

causes detrusor instability; in other children infection may give rise directly to reflux.

Thus the treatment of reflux should be aimed at the triad in Fig. 1.7 and not just the anatomical abnormality.

It is clear that intra-renal reflux plays a very important role in *renal scarring* but at normal voiding pressures sterile intra-renal reflux does not damage kidneys as measured by changes in the glomerular filtration rate (GFR). It is possible, however, that sterile *high* pressure reflux may lead to scarring. However, the pressures needed are those seen in such obstructive conditions as posterior urethral valve or neuropathic bladder. Under normal circumstances, the so-called "water hammer effect" of reflux does not lead to renal scarring. It may result in some tubular damage but, although the abnormalities in tubular function can be detected in children with reflux, scarring does not occur. Another major problem is the distinction between acquired scarring and dysplasia; prenatal diagnosis of reflux will tell more about the natural history of renal scarring. Thus, reflux damages kidneys by means of renal scarring and scarring only occurs when there is a combination of urinary tract infection and intra-renal reflux.

There are many methods of grading reflux but perhaps the most appropriate is the one that was devised by the International Reflux Study Group (Table 1.3). In grade I, reflux enters the lower ureter only, in grade II it fills a non-dilated upper tract. Grades III, IV and V relate to the degree of dilatation and the morphological characteristics such as blunting of the papillae and tortuosity of the ureter. It is often a question of "eye-balling" unless one is involved in the International Reflux Study. It should be noted that it is possible to see reflux and obstruction in the same ureter. An important point to remember is that, in boys, the micturating cystogram should demonstrate the urethra clearly, so that any form of outflow obstruction such as posterior urethral valve is not missed. If the urethra is not demonstrated satisfactorily it may be

Table 1.3. Grading of reflux (International Reflux Study Committee 1981)

Grade I	Reflux into ureter only
Grade II	Reflux to pelvis and calices. No dilatation
Grade III	Mild to moderate dilatation but minimal blunting of calices
Grade IV	Moderate dilatation, loss of angles of fornices
	Papillary impressions in calices still present
Grade V	Gross dilatation and tortuosity. The impressions of the papillae
	are no longer visible

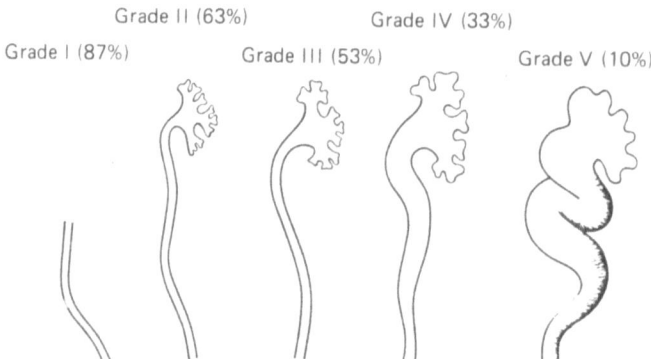

Grade I (87%)   Grade II (63%)   Grade III (53%)   Grade IV (33%)   Grade V (10%)

Fig. 1.8.   Incidence of spontaneous cessation of reflux (Duckett and Bellinger 1984).

necessary to repeat the study. Such reflux which is associated with outflow obstruction is termed "secondary reflux". Other causes of secondary reflux are duplications, bladder diverticulum and neuropathic bladder. An IVU may show the classic appearance of a dysplastic kidney that may be associated with reflux but not caused by it.

Before making any clinical decision it is essential to have some idea of renal parenchymal function. An IVU is rarely good enough for an accurate determination of renal function, particularly as contrast may be refluxing from one ureter into the other. A DMSA scan is essential as the isotope does not appear to any great extent in the filtrate or in the urine after the neonatal period. DMSA can give a quantitative assessment of differential function and is particularly good for demonstrating renal scarring.

The natural history of reflux is of interest. The relative length of the intramural ureter doubles as children grow during the first twelve years of life and this is the basis of conservative management of reflux. A study from Philadelphia shows that the lower grades of reflux have a high tendency to stop spontaneously as a child grows (Fig. 1.8). Another study, from Washington DC, shows that between 60% and 80% of reflux stops spontaneously in non-dilated ureters (Skoog et al. 1987). This figure drops, of course, with more dilated ureters (Grades III to V). In the same study 40% of ureters overall stopped refluxing spontaneously whilst 15% came to surgery. At the time that this cohort was looked at, 35% were still being followed up; amongst this group were children who were asymptomatic and off prophylaxis and who still had reflux. It was felt safe to allow these children to go into young adult life with their reflux persisting.

A British study from Jean Smellie (Smellie et al. 1981), gives the same message. Amongst 111 kidneys followed up for a mean period of 9.4 years there was an 85% spontaneous cessation of reflux in undilated ureters and 41% in dilated ones. Two other points are worth noting. The growth of kidneys is not influenced by the presence or severity of reflux; it is infection and reflux that damage kidneys. There were 2 fresh scars seen in 574 child-years of prophylaxis. So, in summary, the tendency to spontaneous cessation of reflux is the basis of conservative management and, with careful surveillance, it is most unusual to see new or progressive scarring of the kidney.

As far as surgical correction is concerned, there have been several studies such as the one by John Atwell of Southampton (Atwell and Cox 1981), showing good results from surgery. He documented accelerated renal growth on IVU appearances following reimplantation. A study from Guys' Hospital has documented improvement in GFR after surgery (Scott et al. 1986). It should be pointed out, however, that these are uncontrolled studies and it is possible that the same results might be seen after successful medical treatment.

Thus, both medical and surgical treatment can be shown to be effective; but what criteria should be used to decide between the two? There have been several studies comparing medical and surgical treatment, such as the Birmingham reflux study (1987), which was probably the biggest. Children with Grades III and IV reflux were allocated either to operation or to conservative management and the conservatively treated children were compared with those who had successful surgery. After 2 years there was no difference in the GFR, renal growth, the appearance of fresh or progressive scarring or the incidence of break-through infection. Even after a successful reimplantation, the incidence of break-through infection may still be considerable. The problem of dysfunctional voiding remains, therefore.

The authors' pathway for the management of reflux starts with a period of conservative management in virtually every child. If prophylaxis is successful conservative treatment is continued until the child is about 5 years of age, although this age is now being lowered. If a child presents after the age of 5 years, low-dose antibiotics are given for at least one year; it is essential to ensure that the child is emptying his/her bladder satisfactorily and is taking the antibiotics, if the prophylaxis is failing, and if he/she is getting symptomatic infections as opposed to asymptomatic bacteriuria. The plan must, naturally, be altered if there is genuine evidence of failure of prophylaxis and the refluxing ureters are then reimplanted. When a child stops prophylaxis at the age of 5 years, the parents are supplied with an antibiotic to keep at home so that they can treat infection promptly. If after stopping the chemo-prophylaxis the child starts to have further symptomatic infections, the ureter must be reimplanted. This, however, is extremely rare. Occasionally a child may have mild cystitis-type symptoms but this is not an indication for reimplantation. Thus, the indications for surgery are first on a functional basis and second on the way that the children respond to initial treatment. The second group have to be considered on an anatomical basis as there are some that are very unlikely to stop refluxing spontaneously. However, reimplantation is not determined purely on the basis of an anatomical abnormality. For instance, many girls with duplex systems manage perfectly well with conservative treatment.

Trimethoprim is probably the drug of choice for conservative treatment and it can be given as a single night-time dose. It is most important that these girls empty their bladders satisfactorily and a voiding drill is mandatory. If bladder instability is diagnosed the child should be given oxybutynin chloride or another anti-cholinergic drug. It should be emphasised to the parents that the moment that the child has any symptoms, the urine should be checked.

From a surgical point of view there are options other than reimplantation. In a neonate with a large ureter and a small bladder, the upper urinary tract can be defunctioned. In the past this was done by ureterostomy but the same result can now be achieved with a *vesicostomy*. Through a lower abdominal incision, the dome of the bladder is freed and the obliterated umbilical ligaments ligated.

A disc of skin is excised and the fundus is brought out as a cutaneous vesicostomy. All paediatric urologists should consider a vesicostomy instead of ureterostomy in controlling the effect of gross reflux in infants. It does not make the subsequent reimplantation any more difficult: it is unwise to attempt to reimplant a large ureter into a small bladder without considerable experience of this technique.

A vesicostomy in a child with reflux would be useful if there are symptomatic infections that are difficult to control on conservative treatment or where there is reflux into a poorly functioning upper tract. Vesicostomy is preferable to a suprapubic cystostomy as a vesicostomy can be left for a year to 18 months but a suprapubic catheter falls out, gets infected and collects calculus material around it. Vesicostomy is a particularly convenient way of diverting the urine as the urine drains into the nappy in the usual way. It is acceptable to the parents and it usually works well. One of the problems is post-operative oedema of the vesicostomy and a catheter left in for a short time usually helps with this.

There seems little doubt that the Cohen operation has a lot to offer as a method of reimplantation. It is an advancement procedure. The ureter is mobilised intra-vesically and put into a transverse trigonal tunnel. Technically it is a much more satisfactory operation than the Leadbetter. The Leadbetter operation, however, is still sometimes necessary in association with a psoas hitch. The psoas hitch should be mentioned as it is an option sometimes necessary during reimplantation. If one kidney is very poorly functioning it may be best removed and all the effort concentrated on a long reimplantation on the opposite side with a psoas hitch. This allows an extremely long tunnel and is a useful manoeuvre. Alternatively, a trans-uretero-ureterostomy can be performed. One of the problems of the Leadbetter operation was kinking at the site of entry into the bladder, particularly when the bladder is full. A study comparing the various types of reimplantation from Rotterdam (Carpentier et al. 1982), shows that there was a success rate of stopping reflux with the Cohen operation of some 98% compared with 88% by other methods. There were no instances of obstruction using the Cohen method whereas there were three with the Leadbetter operation. Furthermore, these operations were done by the residents as well as the consultants and this is surely the test of a good operation.

Finally, there is the STING, the sub-trigonal injection of Teflon, an operation popularised by Barry O'Donnell in Dublin (O'Donnell and Puri 1986). Teflon paste is injected under the sub-mucosal part of the ureter. The STING is a very effective way of preventing reflux. The potential problem remains the injection of the Teflon itself. Although people have been injecting vocal folds for a number of years, the lymphatic drainage is poor from the vocal folds and it is, of course, being used in adults and not children. There is some concern about the risks of putting Teflon particles into children as they may be there for the next 60–70 years. The paste is a suspension of very small particles of Teflon in glycerine and in experimental animals it is possible to demonstrate Teflon in the lymph nodes and lungs. It may be that when biologically compatible material such as collagen is used, the STING will become a more acceptable procedure.

In summary, renal scarring in most instances is an early event which can rarely be prevented: one way towards prevention would be to try to detect reflux in neonates before the scarring has occurred and when the children are still asymptomatic. Uncomplicated reflux which accounts numerically for the vast majority of children tends to stop spontaneously. Reflux, per se, does not damage kidneys and is probably of less importance in older children. As far as the type of treatment is concerned, one can take one's choice as the various studies that have been published so far are largely inconclusive.

References

Atwell JD, Cox PA (1981) Growth of the kidney following unilateral antireflux surgery. Eur Urol 7: 257–262

Birmingham Reflux Study Group (1987) Prospective trial of operative versus non operative treatment of severe vesico-ureteric reflux in children: five years observation. Br Med J 295: 237–241

Carpentier PJ, Bettink PJ, Hop WCJ, Schroder FH (1982) Reflux – a retrospective study of 100 ureteric reimplantations by the Politano-Leadbetter method and 100 by the Cohen technique. Br J Urol 54: 230–233

Duckett JW, Bellinger MF (1984) Vesicoureteric reflux: A comparison of non-surgical and surgical management. In: Hodson J (ed) Reflux nephropathy update, contributions to nephrology. Karger, Basle pp 81–93

Hanna MK (1984) Occult reflux: a prospective study. Presented at Meeting of the American Urological Association, New Orleans (Abstract 7).

Jenkins GR, Noe HN (1982) Familial vesico-ureteric reflux: a prospective study. J Urol 128: 774–778

Kincaid-Smith P (1983) Reflux nephropathy. Br Med J 286: 2002–2003

Koff SA, Lapides J, Piazza DH (1979) Association of urinary infection and reflux with uninhibited bladder contractions and voluntary sphincter obstruction. J Urol 122: 373–376

McKerrow W, Davidson-Lamb N, Jones PF (1984) Urinary tract infection in children. Br Med J 289: 299–303

O'Donnell B, Puri P (1986) Endoscopic correction of primary vesico-ureteric reflux. Br J Urol 58: 601–604

Scott DJ, Blackford HN, Joyce MRL et al. (1986) Renal function following surgical correction of vesico-ureteric reflux in childhood. Br J Urol 58: 119–124

Skoog SJ, Belman AB, Majd M (1987) A non surgical approach to the management of primary vesico-ureteral reflux. J Urol 138: 941–946

Smellie JM, Edwards D, Normand ICS, Prescod N (1981) Effect of vesico-ureteric reflux on renal growth in children with urinary tract infection. Arch Dis Child 56: 593–600

Snyder H McC (1985) Congenital disorders of the ureter. In: Whitfield HN, Hendry WF (eds) Textbook of genitourinary surgery, 1. Churchill Livingstone, London pp 150–154

Further Reading

Kaplan GW, Packer MG (1988) Surgical management of ureteral duplications. In: King LR (ed) Problems in urology. Developmental anomalies and their management, Vol. 2. Lippencott, Philadelphia, pp 69–80

Kelalis PP (1976) Renal pelvis and ureter. In: Kelalis PP, King LR (eds) Clinical pediatric urology, Chapter 14. Saunders, Philadelphia

Stephens FD (1983) Congenital malformations of the urinary tract. Praeger, New York

Whitaker RH (1979) The classification and management of upper urinary tract duplications. In: Lumley J, Craven J (eds) Surgical review 1. Pitman Medical, Tunbridge Wells, England, pp 267–283

Chapter 2

Is There a Place for Reimplanting Ureters that Reflux?

Robert H. Whitaker and Philip G. Ransley

The decision whether or not to reimplant a ureter with reflux is often a difficult one and is frequently based more on "gut feelings" than on any scientific assessment. It is interesting to ask from basic principles why one should consider reimplanting the ureter. Either one is reimplanting a ureter to prevent scarring of the kidney, which is, of course, a good indication but probably rarely achieved, or one is trying to prevent illness in the child. It seems that, on occasions, one definitely improves the general health of the child with re-implantation of the ureter. Of course, the same improvement in health can be achieved with antibiotics, but they give no guarantee that the reflux will stop whereas, hopefully, after an operation there is a very real chance that the reflux will stop. With antibiotics, when the course is finished, a reimplantation may still be necessary.

Some years ago one would have wondered why it was that one child, after numerous attacks of infection and reflux, had produced no scarring of the kidney whilst another child with similar history and appearances had suffered considerable scarring of the kidney. We know now, of course, that it is the shape of the papilla that matters. It is only with a compound papilla that intra-renal reflux and hence renal scarring can occur. Intra-renal reflux is rarely demonstrated in practice, but when it does occur it is often quite dramatic and, after infection, scarring can be demonstrated on repeated studies. Fig. 2.1 shows a dramatic example of intra-renal reflux with subsequent scarring.

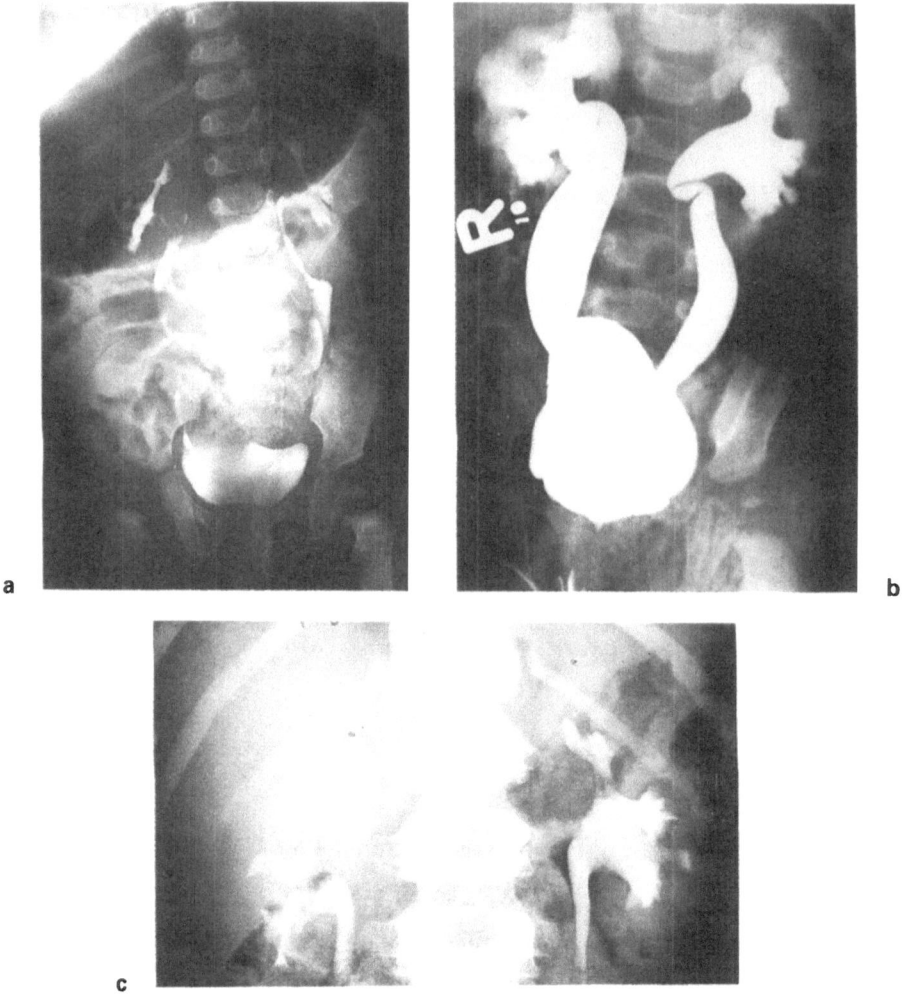

Fig. 2.1a, b, c.   X-rays of a child with severe intra-renal reflux at the age of 6 months. **a.** Initial IVU. No obvious scarring. **b.** Micturating cystogram showing severe intra-renal reflux. **c.** IVU 3 years later showing definite evidence of scarring.

Can We Stop Renal Scarring Occurring?

A paper by Jean Smellie has described 74 children who showed new or progressive renal scarring (Smellie et al. 1987). Although the period over which these children were collected was not given, it was probably in the region of 20 years; the patients came from various centres throughout Great Britain. New or increasing scarring in 34 of these children over the age of 5 years was demonstrated. An estimate of the number of children who were investigated for urinary tract infection over this 20-year-period indicates that something in the region of 50 000 intravenous urograms would be needed to detect these new or progressive scars. This represents one new scar for every 600 IVUs. If the group of children over 5 years old is looked at alone, 1400 IVUs would be needed to detect each new scar. Thus, there is no doubt that Jean Smellie has shown that children's kidneys can develop new scars or increased scarring, but if this is put into perspective with the number of children who are investigated, the numbers really are very small indeed. This suggests that the investigations must be tempered by the likelihood of finding new or increased scarring.

The investigative modalities have been discussed in Chapter 1 and include ultrasound, which can now show the kidney very clearly and can demonstrate abnormalities such as a duplex system with a dilated upper moiety. It is most important with ultrasound that the child has a full bladder, if possible, so that the lower ureters can be inspected behind the bladder. The DMSA scan is still probably the most efficient way of detecting scarring of the kidney and determining differential function. It also shows the anatomy much more clearly in an infant than the IVU; for instance in a horseshoe kidney the isthmus can be delineated accurately. The DTPA scan (Diethylenetriamine penta-acetic acid) is also extremely useful and has largely superceded the IVU in infants with severe impairment of renal function or gross dilatation. In a boy with a posterior urethral valve, DTPA is the investigation of choice.

Investigative Pathways

The flow chart (modified slightly from Whitaker and Sherwood 1987) shows a satisfactory approach to the detection of reflux in small children in whom it might still be possible to detect reflux before scarring has occurred (Fig. 2.2). This applies particularly to children under the age of 3 years. This flow chart also includes investigation of children with an abdominal mass of renal origin and those with haematuria. Thus, in all neonates the investigations that are essential are a plain X-ray examination, an ultrasound of the urinary tract and a micturating cystogram.

The order in which these investigations are performed is not important. In older children, plain X-ray films and ultrasound are all that are needed for the first infection. A micturating cystogram is not performed as an initial investigation in this group because the chance of picking up intra-renal reflux before scarring has occurred in this age group is extremely unlikely. All children with a mass have ultrasound and plain X-ray examinations. If the mass seems to be cystic, a DMSA scintigram is needed to see if there is any function in the kidney. Many of these cystic non-functioning kidneys are multicystic kidneys. A child with a solid mass needs an IVU next and probably a CT scan.

The appearance of a stone on plain X-ray or ultrasound should indicate the need for an IVU, and some other investigation of renal function such as a DTPA scan. If reflux is apparent in the infant on a micturating cystogram, then a DMSA scintigram is necessary at an early stage to detect scarring.

In an older child who has had plain X-ray and ultrasound examinations as the first screening tests for an infection, the result indicates either a normal urinary

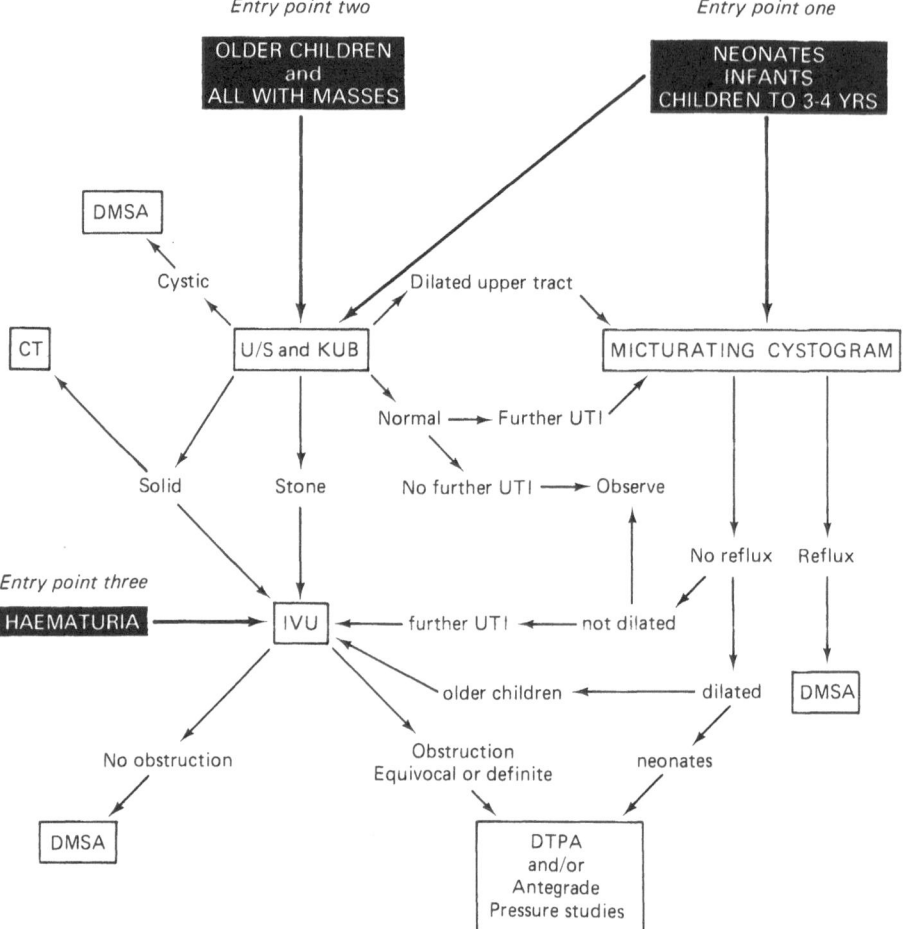

Fig. 2.2. Flow chart for the investigation of children with urinary tract infections. Haematuria and abdominal masses have been included for completeness. (By permission of the Editor of the Lancet, from Whitaker RH, Sherwood T (1987)).

tract or a dilated one. If the urinary tract is normal and the child has no further infection, he can simply be followed up and investigated further as necessary. A further urinary tract infection would probably suggest the need for a micturating cystogram to document reflux and would enable the patient to be treated in the best way in that situation. If the upper urinary tract is dilated on the initial ultrasound, a micturating cystogram would then be indicated to look for reflux. If no reflux is present then the next investigation depends on the age of the child. In a neonate an IVU is probably not the investigation of choice as so much more information is obtained from a DTPA scan. Indeed, it is often an advantage to perform a DMSA scan as well to get additional information. We often perform a percutaneous pressure flow study to look more carefully at the anatomy and measure the pressures to detect obstruction.

In an older child with a dilated non-refluxing upper urinary tract, an IVU is probably the best investigation. In a neonate, in whom the situation is not entirely clear but whose kidneys appear to be functioning adequately, we often wait a month to six weeks and then perform an IVU. At this stage, the infant's kidneys handle the contrast medium much better and useful information is obtained.

In an older child who has had an IVU showing some dilatation, but in whom obstruction is not suspected, it is worth performing a DMSA scan as these children often fit into the category of the pseudo-prune belly syndrome. If some degree of obstruction is suspected, a DTPA scan is helpful and a pressure flow study may give the definitive answer as to the degree of obstruction.

The Relationship between the Number of Previous Infections and Presenting Symptoms, and the Degree of Reflux and the Need for Surgery in Reflux

It has often been suspected that there is little relationship between the severity of the presenting symptoms and the grade of the reflux. At times one sees a child present with severe fever and loin pain; reflux is suspected but a micturating cystogram fails to show it. However, another child ill with mild dysuria has quite severe reflux. A study was recently performed to see if these preconceived ideas are true. From a study of 222 patients with reflux it was found that there was no significant difference in the grading of the reflux or the appearance of renal scars in children who presented with either one or multiple infections (Ozen and Whitaker 1987). This would suggest that severe reflux is as likely to be encountered in a child who has had only one urinary tract infection as in a child who has had multiple infections. It emphasises that the policy of waiting for a second infection before investigating fully is probably not justified.

The symptoms were then classified as mild, moderate or severe according to such factors as mild dysuria, the need to be admitted to hospital and the presence or absence of fever. There was no difference when the severity of symptoms was compared with the degree of scarring and there was virtually no difference when it was compared with the grading of the reflux. Furthermore, in this retrospective study, there was no correlation between the severity of the symptoms and the need for operative intervention. Thus, it would appear that the number or severity of infections bears little relationship to the grading of reflux or the need for operation.

Indications for Reimplanting a Refluxing Ureter

Table 2.1 shows the indications used for reimplanting a refluxing ureter: among them are several physical factors such as the presence of duplications or paraureteral saccule in a boy. Over-distension of the renal pelvis at the height

Table 2.1. Indications for reimplantation of the ureter

---

1. Poor response to adequate medical treatment as shown by break-through infections
2. Inability to tolerate or obtain antibiotics
3. Ballooning of the renal pelvis on micturition
4. Unlikelihood of spontaneous cessation
   certain duplications
   paraureteric saccules in boys
   cystoscopic appearances

Relative indications
5. Gross reflux in early childhood
6. Persistent reflux into puberty
7. Social indications such as the desire of the parents to avoid long-term antibiotics and repeated X-ray examinations or out-patient appointments

---

of voiding on a micturating cystogram would be a factor in favour of reimplanting the ureter. Not everybody would agree that children who are still showing reflux at puberty should have their ureters reimplanted. Fortunately, these children are infrequently seen.

The final factor on the list is perhaps the most contentious. After it has been explained to the parents that there is a 95% chance of the reflux stopping with surgery as compared with a spontaneous cessation rate of approximately 70%, many parents opt for surgical management. The alternative is several more years of antibiotics, micturating cystograms and other investigations whilst, at the end of the day, an operation to reimplant the ureters may still be needed. Just occasionally a family may be moving to live abroad and would rather have the reflux dealt with surgically before they go. Reimplantation is contra-indicated in the presence of chronic renal failure, severe hypertension and very poor ureteric motility.

Technical Considerations

The *Cohen technique* is a very satisfactory method of reimplanting ureters. If both ureters are being reimplanted it is probably best to place one ureter above the other on the trigone. Some surgeons have tried crossing the two ureters over so that the ureteric orifices are more normally placed, but it is doubtful whether this a good plan.

How should wide ureters that need reimplantation be managed? One possibility has been outlined in Chapter 1—a *nephro-ureterectomy* for a poor kidney and a reimplantation of the single ureter. *Trans-uretero-ureterostomy* has also been described with reimplantation of a single ureter. The peritoneum may be removed from the dome of the bladder and both ureters brought across to one side for long sub-mucosal tunnels. The *psoas hitch* operation is a very satisfactory way of fixing the bladder so that the length of the tunnel remains adequate in the post-operative period. The length should always be at least four times the diameter of the ureter. Post-operatively, the psoas hitch certainly distorts the bladder and it probably never empties quite the same again but, in practice, this does not seem to be a practical problem. With the psoas hitch it is, of course, necessary to mobilise the ureter fully both inside and outside the bladder, and bring it down the posterior wall of the bladder with a long sub-mucosal tunnel. It should not be reimplanted through the top of the psoas hitch, but about a centimetre down the posterior wall in case further adjustment is necessary later. The psoas hitch is not a particularly easy procedure as the retroperitoneum needs to be exposed adequately to gain access to the psoas muscle. It is often difficult to get more than one suture into the muscle and care must be taken to avoid including any nerves in the stitch.

What degree of renal failure would dissuade one from reimplanting a ureter? This is to some extent an academic question because the child who presents with severe renal failure often gives no history of urinary tract infections. Such a child presents, perhaps, at the age of 15 years with severe headaches from hypertension and investigations show that there are two small scarred kidneys and severe reflux. The question of reimplanting the ureters to prevent infection does not arise. Thus, one might ask why a reimplantation would be applicable in such a child. Clearly scarring is not going to be prevented, infections are not a problem, and almost certainly a small degree of increased resistance to the flow of urine will be produced. This could represent obstruction for a rather poorly functioning kidney. Some tentative data suggest that renal function can deteriorate after reimplantation in this situation.

An important factor to consider is the possible requirements of a transplant surgeon later. If it is likely that the ureters will be needed at a later date for transplantation purposes then a reimplant might be applicable at this stage. Several years ago, in a small group of children with corrected creatinine clearances between 10 and 15 ml/min, it was found that those children whose ureters had been reimplanted were on dialysis programmes within six months of the reimplantation. Since then, children with this degree of renal failure have not been reimplanted. There is no adequate explanation why reimplantation may precipitate renal failure (Gough, personal communication).

The problem is that the decision was being made on a single investigation. One really needs to know the position of the patient on the slope. For instance, if one looks at boys with posterior urethral valves over a period of time, it often transpires that reimplanting a refluxing ureter does not alter the course of the renal function at all. The data from a trial at The Hospital for Sick Children, Great Ormond Street will soon be analysed after a ten-year follow-up of children with gross bilateral reflux diagnosed under the age of one year. The indications for entry to the trial are shown in Table 2.2. It is a physiological trial that compares successful surgery with successful medical treatment. Success-ful surgery implies getting rid of reflux whereas successful medicine means stopping the urinary tract infections. If either of these treatments failed in either limb, in other words if the medically treated children had break-through

Table 2.2. Criteria for entry to the GOS trial comparing medical with successful surgical treatment

1. Age less than one year
2. Severe bilateral reflux
3. GFR greater than 20 ml/min/1.73 m.sq surface area
4. No abnormal bladder function (outflow obstruction and neuropathic bladder)
5. Adequate follow-up probable
6. Randomisation acceptable

infections or the surgical group were still refluxing, the child was then taken out of the trial. Children with a GFR of less than 20 ml/min were excluded from the trial. Initially, 31 children were considered and 17 were randomised. There were 2 withdrawals from the surgical group, which emphasises the point about the difficulties of reimplanting wide ureters into thin walled bladders in infants, and 4 children were withdrawn from the medical side.

During the first 2 years there was no difference at all between the medical and surgical groups and the natural GFR development occurred in both groups. Using two standard deviations there is no difference between the two groups at 5 years. The completion of the data and publication are awaited. One of the problems of this trial was that the medical group started at a mean overall GFR lower than the surgical group and the question could be asked as to whether hyperfiltration is active in the medical group before it is in the surgical group. Therefore, slight separation between these two groups may be occurring independently of their treatment. This trial is imperfect in that it does not give individual renal function since isotope studies were not available in 1975 when it began, but it does give us confidence that, in the management of even the most severe grades of reflux without outflow obstruction, the child can be managed conservatively during the first two years.

The Conservative Management of Reflux

A few more points about the conservative management of reflux must be emphasised (Table 2.3). Management of the bowel is of paramount importance. Constipation can lead to great problems in the child with reflux. It should be borne in mind that the most common cause of acute urinary retention in young girls is constipation. Dysfunctional voiding is also an important factor and all children with reflux should probably have urodynamic studies. Although the mechanisms are unknown, children with unstable bladders are more liable to urinary tract infections. A topic for debate at the present time in the USA is whether the presence of the foreskin in a young boy makes him more prone to urinary tract infections. A rise in the incidence of *Proteus* urinary tract infection has been noted since routine circumcision was abandoned. Another factor in girls is the use of bubble baths. As the girl plays in the bath she almost certainly sucks some water into her vagina and hence into the bladder; the chemical irritants in bubble baths may be enough to induce cystitis. These other factors must be considered before giving prophylactic antibiotics.

Table 2.3. Conservative management of reflux

Regular voiding
Correction of constipation
Control of instability
Perineal/preputial cleanliness
Avoidance of bubble baths
Reduction of anxiety
Low dose antibiotics at night

A child with reflux may be managed in the following way. Investigation begins when the child is first seen, usually in the first few years of life, with a contrast cystogram and a DMSA scan. Some of these children need primary surgical treatment, for instance those with primary vesico-ureteric pathology in association with reflux, and also those with reflux plus obstruction or with a big baggy paraureteral saccule. The remaining children are put on prophylaxis and the next investigations are planned after 2 years. By that time some of the children will have stopped refluxing. At 2 years they are investigated with a *direct* isotope cystogram. It cannot be an indirect isotope study because the children are still too young at this age to cooperate adequately, but it does not need to be a contrast study; a repeat DMSA scan is also performed at this stage. Some children need reimplantation of the ureter at this stage because of repeated symptomatic break-through infections despite treatment of constipation, oxybutynin chloride for unstable bladder, avoiding bubble baths, etc. Symptomatic urinary tract infections are not necessarily stopped by reimplanting the ureters, but the reimplant may protect the kidney from infection. There may also be social reasons at this stage for reimplanting the ureters: there is some place also for reimplanting ureters in the dysfunctional group as the dysfunction may not respond to treatment but at least the reflux can be abolished.

The second period of follow-up is after a further 3 years, when the child is 5 years old; by that time more ureters will have stopped refluxing. Further studies are performed 5 years from the time that the child was first seen. Prophylactic antibiotics are stopped 6 months before these studies so that by the time the investigations are performed it will be clear whether the child can manage to avoid infections without prophylaxis. An indirect isotope cystogram can now be used and a further DMSA scan is needed. The decision to reimplant the ureter at this stage is based on the presence of symptomatic urinary tract infections. This scheme saves a great deal of thought and agonising decisions over individual patients in out-patients, and is a reasonable approach to reflux given our present level of knowledge.

There is a very real place for reimplanting the ureters of a child who is on intermittent catheterisation for a poorly emptying bladder at the end of the first 6 months of intermittent catheterisation if the reflux is still present. Some of these children on intermittent catheterisation do have high end-filling pressures. In a proportion of these children, of course, the reflux will have stopped after a period of regular intermittent catheterisation.

The management of a child with a pelvi-ureteric obstruction in the presence of reflux depends on the results of an IVU and a micturating cystogram. If the IVU shows no evidence of hydronephrosis or suggestion of pelvi-ureteric obstruction, but the cystogram shows considerable reflux which distends the renal pelvis, then the operation that is needed is reimplantation. At the other end of the scale is the child with hydronephrosis, suggestive of pelvi-ureteric obstruction on the IVU, who also happens, on a micturating cystogram, to have some reflux. The operation in this situation is a pyeloplasty. There is a third group of children who have moderate hydronephrosis on an IVU and moderate reflux on a cystogram. Choosing the correct operation is sometimes difficult. On occasions, both a reimplant and a pyeloplasty can be performed during the same operation as there is no worry about the blood supply in this situation. The alternative is to perform a pyeloplasty first, since obstruction damages a kidney faster and more severely than does reflux in this situation. The infections associated with reflux can be kept in control with antibiotics until a decision is made at a later date as to whether a reimplantion should also be performed.

In the management of the child whose reimplantation has failed the first thing is to look back and make sure that the initial indication to reimplant was correct and to assess whether there were any other factors involved. Once the decision has been made to re-reimplant a ureter then the surgical technique is probably little different from a classical first-time reimplantation. It is always important to make sure that neuropathic bladder or posterior urethral valve has been excluded. Re-reimplantation with a psoas hitch and a trans uretero-ureterostomy above it can be most helpful.

A DMSA scan is a much more accurate way of assessing scarring in kidneys than an IVU, but a number of the studies that have been described have been based on IVU evidence and not on a DMSA scan. Many of them are probably suspect because they do not have the availability of a DMSA scan. This is particularly true in the USA where they have been very slow in accepting its use. It is probably fair to say that the defects seen on the DMSA scan within a short time of the infection are perfusion defects. However, if these perfusion defects are followed up over the months they do seem to correlate very well with the eventual sites of true renal scarring. This would suggest that early changes on a DMSA scan are probably meaningful in terms of predicting eventual scarring.

Urodynamic studies have proved to be useful in children with non-neuropathic problems. The documentation of instability is most important, as is that of obstruction, if one regards bladder sphincter dyssynergia as an obstructive problem. Some of these children present between the ages of 2 years and 3 years with infections. There are two groups of children with reflux; there is a group with a congenital short tunnel that are born with reflux, and there is a second group of children who present at the time of toilet training with some form of transient bladder dysfunction, that may last for months or a few years, who begin refluxing as a result of this poor bladder behaviour. This group may possibly be at a greater risk of acquired renal scarring because of the abnormal bladder behaviour. They also have the highest chance of losing their reflux spontaneously if bladder behaviour can be controlled.

References

Ozen HA, Whitaker RH (1987) Does the severity of presentation in children with vesicoureteric reflux relate to the severity of the disease or the need for operation? Br J Urol 60: 110–112
Smellie JM, Ransley PG, Normand ICS, Precod N, Edwards D (1987) Development of new renal scars: a collaborative study. Br Med J 290: 1957–1960
Whitaker RH, Sherwood T (1987) Diagnostic pathways. Lancet 1: 1266

Further Reading

Corkery JJ (1988) Reimplantation—which child? In: Gingell C, Abrams P (eds) Controversies and
    innovations in urological surgery, Chapter 41. Springer-Verlag, Heidelberg
Ransley PG (1982) Vesicoureteric reflux. In: Williams DI, Johnston JH (eds) Paediatric urology,
    2nd edn. Butterworths, London
Whitaker RH (1988) Reimplantation—which operation? In: Gingell C, Abrams P (eds) Controver-
    sies and innovations in urological surgery, Chapter 42. Springer-Verlag, Heidelberg

Chapter 3

Prune, Pseudo Prune and Other Dysplastic Uropathies

Philip G. Ransley

We are about to witness a revolution in our understanding of dysplastic uropathies. It may become necessary to rewrite some of the previously written chapters on the dilated urinary tract in the infant and the neonate so the dysplastic uropathies mentioned in the title of this chapter make the basis of an interesting discussion. The classic theories of renal dysplasia are no longer tenable.

The word dysplasia is a little like junk food. It is a satisfying word for a short period of time and it gets you out of the immediate problem. However, it does you no good and you swear that you will never use it again, but you find yourself going back to using the term time and time again since there really is no better alternative.

Dysplasia versus Obstruction

The Douglas Stephens theory of dysplastic renal development is familiar to all urologists. The ureteric bud leaves its abnormal origin and hits a bad bit of metanephric blastema which in turn leads to the formation of a dysplastic kidney. This is primary dysplastic development. However, there is experimental evidence that early intrauterine obstruction can also cause dysplastic renal development (Beck 1971; Tanagho 1972). For example, dysplastic kidneys are found in other cases of renal obstruction, such as in boys with a posterior urethral valve who were obstructed in utero. The prune belly baby often has dysplastic kidneys and obstruction may be one of the elements of the prune belly syndrome. However, there is a large group of non-obstructed urinary tracts with dysplastic kidneys which are labelled as "dysplasia". Like junk food the term does not help and it does no good.

It is possible that there may be a transient period of intrauterine obstruction which causes changes in the kidney similar to those seen in dysplasia. By birth, the obstruction is no longer present and the two conditions are then indistinguishable. It would then be impossible to distinguish between primary dysplasia and dysplasia secondary to obstruction. The purpose of this introduction is to stress the need for making a satisfactory diagnosis which is so important if the correct treatment and prognosis are to be given.

In a boy who has had a posterior urethral valve destroyed 3 months previously there is often a dysplastic non-functioning kidney on one side and a better kidney on the opposite, non-refluxing side. A micturating cystogram will show small bilateral para-ureteral diverticula, a nice urethra with good flow and a smooth walled bladder; there is clearly nothing to be done here surgically. The non-refluxing system could be perfused by the Whitaker technique (Whitaker 1979) when it will be shown to be non-obstructive. This diagnosis can be made with confidence and the treatment determined, because the natural history of progress in these boys with a valve, and the necessary follow-up studies, are known.

Alternatively, a child with a smooth-walled bladder on a cystogram should be considered. There is a little hypertrophy of the bladder neck and a dilated posterior urethra but the child is doing well. There is a stable urinary tract with some renal dysplasia. There is reflux into a big ballooned pelvis with short, wide-necked calices and widely dilated and tortuous ureters. Renal dysmorphism is probably a better term here. In this case, we are not so secure clinically because this child did not have a posterior urethral valve as far as we can tell. The insecurity is, to some extent, due to the fact that the urethra is similar to that seen in a child who has had previous obstruction. If there has been obstruction in this child, it must have occurred before birth. The child, in fact, had been found to have an abnormal urinary tract on a prenatal ultrasound and was investigated further soon after birth. Thus, there is an abnormal urinary tract, of uncertain origin. There is no true diagnosis and no reasonable prognosis. Indeed it is not known how to treat such a child. This uncertainty has, at times in the past, lead to unnecessary aggressive surgery in a number of such children. A DMSA scan shows that the kidneys are functioning poorly right from the outset. One is unable to tell at this point whether those abnormal dysplastic kidneys and dysmorphic upper tracts are the consequences of primary ureteric bud maldevelopment, a transient intrauterine problem which has now resolved, or simple reflux which may be a continuing problem as far as the kidneys are concerned. This type of case may well represent a transient intrauterine obstruction which has resolved, leaving the child with a dysplastic urinary tract which is now in a stable state. Such cases have been seen many times over the years and the tendency has been to dismiss them as dysplastic systems without considering the possibility of intrauterine obstruction.

A further example, which reinforces the belief that these changes may be due to transient intrauterine obstruction, can be given. The mother of a male fetus had a prenatal fetal ultrasound at 21 weeks of gestation which showed a distended bladder with bilateral hydroureteronephrosis but a normal amount of amniotic fluid. At 25 weeks gestation the bladder was noted to be full, there was still mild hydronephrosis and still a normal amount of amniotic fluid. At 26 weeks the bladder was seen to be enormous and varied in volume between 48 and 60 ml on ultrasound. This is large for a baby of 26 weeks gestation. A little later there was evidence of oligohydramnios with increasing hydronephrosis. A short time later, mother and fetus were readmitted to hospital with a view to placement of a shunt and repeat ultrasound showed that the bladder was now empty but thick-walled. There was still moderate hydronephrosis but the quantity of amniotic fluid had returned to normal. These appearances remained constant through to term as one would expect after decompression of the bladder. After birth the child passed urine satisfactorily. The cystogram showed para-ureteral diverticula, posterior bladder neck hypertrophy and an abnormal, slightly dilated posterior urethra. The child continues to void satisfactorily, empties the bladder completely and has not undergone a cystoscopy. This case illustrates the possibility of transient intrauterine obstruction as a cause of an otherwise inexplicable dysplastic urinary tract. Such cases may not be rare and more will be seen as they are searched for.

The non-refluxing non-obstructed megaureter has been a source of anxiety for many years. It is difficult to imagine how, in a unilateral case, the ureter could become so dilated unless there was a true obstruction at the lower end of the ureter. One explanation is that the child had a posterior urethral valve causing a transient intrauterine obstruction and this caused reflux into the system that is now dilated. As is seen so often after relief of valve obstruction, the reflux stops spontaneously. Had we seen this appearance in a boy with a posterior urethral valve in whom we had resected the valve ourselves, we would be comfortable with it. However, when we see the case de novo, we are uncomfortable because we do not know exactly what happened. I believe we should look for transient prenatal obstruction as an explanation for some of these problems.

Prune Belly Syndrome

There seems little doubt that the classical "prune" is an acquired disorder. The prune belly syndrome is the most florid example of the dysplastic uropathies and merits brief discussion. One feature of the prune is the absence of the abdominal wall muscles; this can be shown to be a non-specific response to gross abdominal distension in utero. Absent or poor abdominal musculature is occasionally seen in other conditions such as posterior urethral valves, Hirschsprung's disease, and in children with tumours occupying the abdominal cavity. Any form of abdominal distension can cause a prune belly. The timing of the distension is critical if it is to influence embryological events such as the movement of mesoderm around to form the abdominal wall.

There may be a galaxy of different urethral problems which can give rise to massive urinary tract dilatation. These problems may last for different lengths of time, and may be of different degrees of severity so that the combination of severity, type, timing of onset and duration may all affect what the dysplastic uropathy and other abnormalities become. The prune belly syndrome is probably just one of these abnormalities and it is clear from prenatal ultrasound studies and the subsequent abortion or delivery of children that the urinary tract becomes distended very early during development in the prune belly syndrome. Thus, the absent abdominal wall, intra-abdominal testes and other urinary tract abnormalities make up the prune belly syndrome. The urinary tract abnormalities include renal dysplasia, dilated tortuous ureters, an enormous bladder and an abnormal urethra. The abnormal urethra in its most serious form is a complete atresia which may or may not be associated with a patent urachus. Other abnormalities of the urethra include megalourethra and extreme flaccidity of the abdominal wall so that it flops over in the most extraordinary way taking the guts with it. There is often a small mark on the lower abdominal wall and dimples on the knees and elbows in boys with prune belly syndrome. If the child is seen in the first few hours after birth, these areas may be raw and if the legs and arms are folded up, the knees or heels fit into these spots. They are a secondary indication of intrauterine compression. Douglas Stephens believes that even some forms of hypospadias are associated with the child's heel pressing into the perineum.

The Urethra in the Prune Belly Syndrome

A cystogram in the typical prune belly child shows a very large bladder which flops forward, a distal megalourethra and a narrowing in the posterior urethra

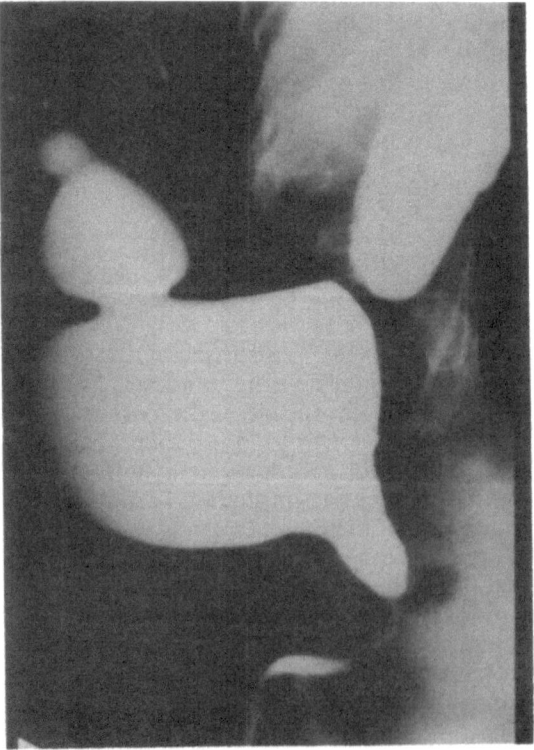

Fig. 3.1.   Micturating cystogram of a child with prune belly syndrome. Note the dilated urethra.

with proximal elongation and ballooning (Fig. 3.1). It is often difficult to decide the level of the bladder neck. Although Fig. 3.1 is a cystogram, this investigation is probably the one thing not to do in the prune child in the neonatal period because of the extremely high risk of introducing infection. With infection and a bladder capacity of over 200 ml, these children can become extremely sick. In addition, there is often a urachal remnant in these children, perhaps in the form of urachal cyst above the bladder. There may or may not be reflux into grossly dilated and tortuous ureters. To reiterate, the prune abnormality probably lies in the posterior urethra, although nobody has, as yet, successfully documented this abnormality. It is not a valve and whatever it is, it is difficult to identify endoscopically. In these children there is a narrowing in the posterior urethra on voiding, that can undoubtedly cause a degree of outflow obstruction. In addition, they have poor detrusor activity. The dome of the bladder in a prune belly syndrome is almost completely devoid of muscle and does not contract. In contrast, the lower half of the bladder, particularly the bladder base, has well-preserved muscle in it and can contract adequately. Thus, when a prune belly bladder tries to empty itself it does so in three ways. Urine is expelled down the urethra, into one or other of the ureters by reflux, and into the dome of the bladder which is unable to contract. A cystogram shows the urine going in all three directions, but only a small proportion of urine passes down the urethra. The appearance of the prune urethra is often one of tapering down to the narrow segment.

Management of Prune Belly Syndrome

The management of the prune is essentially conservative except for the urethra. The grossly dilated upper tracts and bladder may do extremely well on conservative management. Sometimes the only treatment that is necessary is an internal urethrotomy through the narrowed area. Attention must be devoted to making sure that the bladder empties as best it can. Continence does not seem to be a problem after internal urethrotomy in these children. It must be emphasised that only committed paediatric urologists dealing regularly with the prune syndrome in established units should operate on these children. The urethrotomy is done in the twelve o'clock position right through from the bladder neck down to and entering the external sphincter. The abnormal segment lies within the external sphincter and the distal urethral mechanism. One probably needs to enter this area to obtain satisfactory resolution. If a minor degree of wetting is induced by an internal urethrotomy in these children, this is not too important because such minor degrees almost always improve with time. The internal urethrotomy should not be too radical on the first occasion. It is a simple matter to repeat it, cutting gently each time, and two or three attempts may be needed to get it right. Once the bladder empties satisfactorily the situation usually remains stable and there is a general tendency to improve. The internal urethrotomy should not be performed in infants as it is probably rarely needed in that age group, and is technically most difficult at this age.

The prune belly syndrome illustrates the presence of a posterior urethral obstruction which is sometimes complete, sometimes partial, and sometimes transient but not valvular; we have recognised and talked about this aspect of the condition for some years but we have not applied it until more recently.

This discussion of obstruction is really about relative obstruction. The same degree of narrowing in any other child would probably be insignificant. Here, the child has a very large, poorly contracting bladder and a urethral resistance which is probably entirely normal if compared with normal children but, in the prune belly syndrome, the resistance must be reduced to an abnormally low level so that this poorly contractile bladder can cope. Thus, if one regards obstruction as a high pressure, low flow problem, then the narrowing in the prune belly syndrome cannot be regarded as an obstruction. The situation is managed in the same way as any child with a large poorly contracting bladder would be managed, without the use of intermittent catheterisation. Internal urethrotomy must remain a central consideration in the management of these children.

Undescended Testes in Prune Belly Syndrome

The final problem to discuss in the management of the prune belly syndrome is that of the undescended testes which are intra-abdominal. It is always said that they are intra-abdominal as a result of the other problems of the syndrome and are not dysgenetic. As a consequence it is appropriate to attempt to place such testes in the scrotum, which may be best achieved by a two-stage Fowler–Stephens orchidopexy. This involves an initial ligation of the gonadal vessels, followed by an interval of time for the collateral circulation to develop through the vas. At a second stage the testis is moved down to the scrotum on the vasal vessels. This technique has given extremely good results in the management of the testis in the prune belly syndrome and is now often used as the primary treatment. There is only one recorded testicular tumour in a 25-year-old prune belly syndrome boy who had had three previous orchidopexies on the same testis, the testis not reaching the scrotum until the age of 15 years.

One of the traditional ways of managing a boy with the prune belly syndrome was to perform high ureterostomies, but there are a number of reasons for avoiding these, the most important of which is that ureterostomy, especially a ring ureterostomy, uses up a lot of the ureter. The upper ureter in these children is the best bit of ureter and thus one does not want to use it up performing a ureterostomy. If for some reason a ureterostomy becomes mandatory, bilateral end-ureterosotomies disconnecting them from the bladder wall and bringing them out as a single stoma may be done in such a way that the lower ureter is not excised. Thus, we would have available the full length of the ureter for later reconstruction. High ureterostomies performed in the past caused considerable difficulties with subsequent surgical reconstruction and we have now abandoned these procedures.

Thus, a scheme for the management of the child with prune belly syndrome may be summarised. One is asked to see the child soon after birth. Nothing active should be done at this stage. Renal function is assessed with serial creatinine estimations. The child will be born, of course, with a creatinine which reflects the level in the mother of approximately 80 mgm% to 100 mgm%. In those children with dysplastic kidneys and poor renal function, the creatinine will climb in the first days after birth, but will ultimately plateau off some time up to the sixth day, the level depending upon the GFR. Just because the creatinine is climbing it does not mean that there is a problem within the urinary tract that needs urgent action.

It is important to watch and see whether the child voids urine through the urethra or whether it leaks from a patent urachus. Alternatively, the urine may be coming from a vesicocutaneous double J tube which has been inserted prenatally. Recently in a child born with a double J, there was satisfactory drainage for the first 3 or 4 weeks after birth without any problem. Investigations at this stage should include ultrasound. Provided there are no other abdominal or respiratory problems, ultrasound is all that is needed: a cystogram should not be performed. Provided that urine is draining from somewhere, the child can be left alone until about 1 month of age. Then the kidneys should be assessed with a DMSA scan and a micturating cystogram performed under gentamycin cover. Renal function is again assessed.

In those children who have very poor renal function and in those with a large volume of residual urine, vesicostomy is the best solution. This provides the best possible urinary drainage in the first year of life and allows renal function to develop as best it can. If the child gets into trouble in the first few days of life then a vesicostomy would be appropriate and this can be performed even without a cystogram. If and when the vesicostomy is necessary it is a good opportunity to ligate the testicular vessels on each side as the first stage of the orchidopexy. The vesicostomy can be left for at least 12–18 months. During that time renal function should be assessed regularly.

At the end of this time the aim is to restore urinary tract continuity via a laparotomy with a big "smile" incision. The vesicostomy should be closed with a suprapubic catheter in place. A bilateral Fowler–Stephens orchidopexy is performed together with abdominal wall reduction or plication. The late chest problems in these children, which can be quite considerable, are of interest. All the children have flared ribs when they are born. The ribs may even turn upwards from the junction at the spine producing a relative, rather than a true pectus excavatum.

Tightening up the abdominal wall may put tension on the lower ribs and sternum to lessen these abnormalities. Following reconstruction, the child should have a repeat cystogram to see how well the bladder empties. Thereafter, internal urethrotomy is performed, if necessary, with a suprapubic catheter in place, to establish satisfactory voiding. The suprapubic catheter is then removed. This effort to establish satisfactory voiding is the main feature of management during this follow-up period. Thus, it should be emphasised that there is no rush in the initial treatment of these children nor should a cystogram be performed. Most other things can be achieved under two or three anaesthetics during the first three years of life.

References

Beck AD (1971) The effect of intrauterine urinary obstruction upon the development of the fetal kidney. J Urol 105: 784–789

Tanagho EA (1972) Surgically induced partial urinary obstruction in the fetal lamb. Invest Urol 10: 25–34

Whitaker RH (1979) The Whitaker test. Urol Clin North Am 6: 529–539

Further Reading

Duckett JW (1976) The prune belly syndrome. In: Kelalis PP, King LR (eds) Clinical paediatric
    urology, Chapter 16. Saunders, Philadelphia
Stephens FD (1983) Congenital malformations of the urinary tract. Praeger, New York

Chapter 4

Genito-urinary Tumours in Children

David C. S. Gough

Many urologists find it difficult to keep up-to-date with the management of genito-urinary tumours in children because the methods of management that have been described are so complex and are modified frequently.

Wilms' Tumour (Nephroblastoma)

The vast majority of children with Wilms' tumour are dealt with by paediatric oncologists, but despite this it is still primarily a surgical problem: in my practice, it remains the most common cause of an abdominal mass in children (Table 4.1).

Table 4.1. Malignant abdominal masses in children (Royal Manchester Children's Hospital 1985)

Wilms' tumour	4
Neuroblastoma	3
Rhabdomyosarcoma	1
Pelvic teratoma	1
Adrenal carcinoma	1
Non-Hodgkins lymphoma	1

The first investigation is usually intravenous urography which shows the typical appearances of displaced calices indicating the presence of a Wilms' tumour. There are, however, some traps for the unwary. In order to get the maximum information from the X-ray films it is important for the radiologist to be aware of the clinical problem. There may be variable dilatation of the pelvi-caliceal system from compression by the tumour mass. The tumour has been frequently misdiagnosed in the past. The first MRC study in the UK showed that 3% of the children undergoing surgery had an inappropriate initial operation for what was thought to be an obstructed hydronephrosis. No doubt these problems will continue to arise and we will be caught out from time to time.

It is important to feel the mass and correlate it with the X-ray findings. There are one or two other conditions which can be confusing and mimic a Wilms' tumour in a small child. Sometimes a large abdominal swelling is associated with some degree of distortion of the caliceal pattern on IVU, which may indicate a multilocular cyst (cystic nephroma) of the kidney. In this particular condition the treatment is nephrectomy as it is almost impossible to distinguish the normal from the abnormal renal tissue. It is one of several benign conditions that can give a renal mass (Table 4.2).

Table 4.2. Benign abdominal masses in children (Royal Manchester Children's Hospital 1985)

Multicystic kidney	2
Xanthogranulomatous pyelonephritis	1
Hepatic hamartoma	1
Hepatic haemangioma	1
Lymphangioma of bowel	1
Sacrococcygeal teratoma	2

Table 4.3. Improvement in 3-year disease-free survival for Wilms' tumour (%). Note that no treatment at all is fatal. (Multiple reference sources)

1920	15
1950	34
1960	48
1970	54
1980	77
1986	85

A multicystic kidney is probably the most common mass, but many of these are now being confidently diagnosed prenatally. Xanthogranulomatous pyelo-nephritis is nearly always associated with a non-functioning kidney. The child presents with a long history of illness with a high ESR, a low haemoglobin, low plasma proteins and a non-functioning kidney which is palpable in the loin.

The reason that surgeons in the UK and in the USA have adopted a policy of initial laparotomy and subsequent chemotherapy is because those in the European Wilms' study group (SIOP–Societie Internationale Oncologie Paedi-atrique) treat patients with chemotherapy before surgery and have inevitably treated some 5% of patients with potentially toxic drugs for what transpired to be benign conditions. A histological diagnosis is sought before chemotherapy in the UK and the USA.

There has been an enormous improvement in the outcome of children with Wilms' tumour over the last 60 years (Table 4.3). The first effective treatment for Wilms' tumour was surgical treatment; before this, all children with this condition died. Wilms' tumour is always progressive, albeit sometimes slowly. The early descriptions suggested that some of these children slowly died over a period of nine months or a year with cachexia, increasing abdominal mass and pulmonary secondaries. In the early days, some did not survive the operation. By the 1920s a series of surgical removal alone showed a long-term survival of 15%. A little later, when radiotherapy was added to the surgery, the survival rate rose, in the best centres, to approximately 50%; however, a 33% survival was more usual.

It was in 1956, when D'Angio was able to obtain the drug Actinomycin D and to use it in children with Wilms' tumour, that a further dramatic improvement in survival occurred, such that over half the patients were consistently surviving with a combination of surgery, radiotherapy and Actinomycin D. Since then there have been many other chemotherapeutic drugs used and much more is known about the natural history of the condition. As a result the survival rate in the last decade has been in the region of 85%.

Prior to chemotherapy metastases caused death. Chemotherapy can now control these metastases and has led to the major increase in survival. However, the effects of chemotherapy and radiotherapy are not always beneficial. Radiotherapy to the renal fossa can cause growth defects with permanent scoliosis. Many of these children are also sterile. This is the price that one pays for this type of treatment.

Staging of Wilms' Tumour

Stage 1 is a small intra-renal tumour. Stage 2 is where the renal capsule is penetrated by tumour but is completely removed. Stage 3 is when it seems that the whole tumour has been removed, but it has not. It may have ruptured intraperitoneally either during the operation or perhaps before it, or there are lymph node metastases. There is often some confusion as to the true definition of the Stage 3 Wilms' tumour, which is a histological staging essentially of microscopic disease. Stage 4 disease is clearly not curable surgically because there are metastases at presentation, usually in the lung as well as tumour in the kidney. Stage 5 is bilateral tumour at presentation.

Review of Treatment

Four of the main trials of chemotherapy over the last fifteen years have been reviewed. They all looked at different areas of chemotherapy asking the questions "How much do you have to give?" "How often do you have to give it?" and "How long do you have to give it?" The first MRC study in the UK was designed to show whether Vincristine was better than Actinomycin D and it showed that it was better in Stage 1 disease. Estimation of how long the drug should be given showed that a short course of 6 months in Stage 1 disease was just as good as a long course. Thus, these trials showed that Vincristine was an effective drug in Stage 1 disease and that it was only needed for 6 months. All the National Wilms' Tumour Studies (NWTS) trials used a combination of Vincristine and Actinomycin D. The results of these trials confirmed that it is not necessary to give the two drugs together and that Vincristine was the better drug, which could be used alone. In Stage 1 disease there is no need to give radiotherapy. Thus, for Stage 1 disease only one drug is needed and that is Vincristine for 6 months, with subsequent trials suggesting a reduction to 3 months.

If Stage 4 tumours that present with metastases in the lung, bones or liver are considered, it is seen that these tumours were uniformly fatal until combination chemotherapy was available. Chemotherapy can now save most of these children unless there are metastases in the bones. No child has yet survived with a metastatic Wilms' tumour in bone.

Surprisingly, treatment for Stage 5 disease, bilateral at the time of presentation, is more effective than for Stage 4 disease. In fact, the majority of patients with Stage 5 disease do remarkably well with an 80% 3-year survival. The treatment for Stage 5 disease is nephrectomy for the worst side and partial nephrectomy for the less affected side. If the whole tumour cannot be removed it is worth giving local radiation and chemotherapy and some of these children have survived. In no other stage of Wilms' tumour have patients survived if the tumour has not been removed surgically. If a nephrectomy has not been performed with total removal of the tumour there have been no reported cases of survival in Stages 1 to 4, but there are survivors with Stage 5 disease after known incomplete surgical removal. Thus, the message seems to be that one does not attempt to do "bench surgery" or take out both kidneys and put the patient onto dialysis and a transplantation programme. The best overall results seem to have come from major tumour resection, but leaving enough renal tissue for survival.

If the treatment for Wilms' tumour is so successful, why do patients still die? Persistent disease is the cause of death in 15% of patients, and 3%–5% die as a result of treatment. The results of various British studies show that one-third of patients with renal tumours are not treated in a major oncological centre. In other countries, such as India, the majority of patients present with advanced disease and non-function of the kidney. It must be remembered that these European figures show the best that can be achieved and that, overall, results are not generally successful. In a series of 50 cases followed up for 3 years it was found that one patient died because of the operation, 8 developed recurrent tumours of which 7 were lung metastases and these all died. One patient developed a metachronous tumour in the opposite kidney, had a partial nephrectomy and went through a period of acute renal failure, but then fully recovered with no sign of disease. Thus it can be seen that children who do badly usually develop metastases in the lungs and, in general, these tumours cannot be treated adequately.

In most major series there is a 1%–2% mortality for the operation and perhaps twice that mortality for the chemotherapy itself; this mortality from chemotherapy is not always from the high dose treatment that is given for a relapse (Table 4.4). Death during surgery is nearly always due to tumour embolus, but may result from post-operative haemorrhage. In one case in the British series, a child had the opposite renal artery ligated during initial surgery and this subsequently led to death. The child had a period of dialysis and an unsuccessful kidney transplant but died 6 months later. Tumour embolus occurs when there is major involvement of the vena cava evident before operation. Nowadays most paediatric urologists would want to be sure that there is no caval extension before embarking upon a primary nephrectomy. If

Table 4.4. Death associated with treatment of Wilms' tumour (SIOP)

Surgery	1%–2%
Chemotherapy/DXT	2%[a]
(as initial treatment)	
Chemotherapy/DXT	0.75%
(for relapse disease)	

[a]Stage of disease: no. of deaths. 1:1, 2:6,
3:1, 4:2

intracaval tumour is present, the patient would be treated with chemotherapy
before an attempt was made to remove the tumour.

How careful should one be when taking out the renal tumour? One of the
reasons why the SIOP studies were started was because it was shown that
intra-operative rupture of the tumour during removal worsened the prognosis.
There was a slight increase in the overall mortality. Those carrying out the
SIOP study then decided that they must take every possible precaution to avoid
intra-operative rupture: they decided upon pre-operative treatment which
involves Vincristine therapy and has now reduced their intra-operative rupture
rate to 3%. The majority of surgeons outside SIOP find that 16%–20% of
tumours rupture at the time of operation. It is possible to reduce this rate
somewhat by careful surgery, but probably not down to the level reached in the
SIOP studies.

It is necessary to remove some glands from around the aorta for subsequent
pathological staging. It is not good enough simply to look at the nodes; they
must be biopsied. A major lymphadenectomy, however, is not necessary. It is
interesting to note that one of the post-operative complications is intussuscep-
tion. Obstruction from adhesions is a very real problem, but it does not always
require a further laparotomy. Some of the children develop a hydrocele on
long-term follow-up.

The first basic principle of the management of Wilms' tumour, therefore, is to
make sure that the tumour is completely removed at the first operation. In
Stage 1 disease with favourable histology it is not even necessary to give
Vincristine for 6 months. The treatment with Vincristine can be for just 12
weeks only. The chances of survival with favourable histology in Stage 1 is
about 99%. In Stage 2, where the tumour has been completely removed and the
lymph nodes are negative, the children are given Vincristine and Actinomycin
D; the chances of success are high and the risks of recurrent tumour in the
abdomen are low. In Stage 3, three drugs are necessary. A further guiding
principle is that all efforts should be made to avoid tumour embolus. Despite all
this care, all children with Wilms' tumours will not be cured. Unfortunately
some children will still succumb from the chemotherapy (2%) and others from
persistent or recurrent tumour, (12%–14%).

A very large renal tumour can be treated primarily with chemotherapy; the
mass completely shrinks away, but the question remains of whether it is still
necessary to remove the diseased kidney. Nobody has survived after leaving a
tumour in situ, but there have been no formal trials of leaving the kidney in
place in this situation. Results from successful removal of the kidney are
excellent, so it would perhaps be difficult to justify this conservative approach.

In most trials the protocol provides that the other kidney must be exposed and inspected but it is only rarely that such tumour is found in these circumstances. It has been reported that a tumour has been found on the posterior surface of the opposite kidney that had not been detected by any diagnostic modality. The tumour was about 1 cm in diameter (Ransley, personal communication). Ransley suggests that both surfaces of the opposite kidney should be routinely inspected before attempting to remove the diseased kidney: if a tumour is seen in the opposite kidney, or if one is known to be present from previous diagnostic studies, that tumour and the main tumour in the opposite kidney are both biopsied and the patient is closed without removal of the main diseased kidney. This is because Ransley has found on two occasions that the small tumour in the contra-lateral kidney has unfavourable histology and it would have been more appropriate to leave in the kidney with the large tumour and more favourable histology. With bilateral disease his policy now is biopsy only and subsequent chemotherapy. Once the lesions have shrunk, some form of conservative surgical treatment can be considered. Furthermore, the possibility of a more conservative approach in Stage 4 after chemotherapy to the question of whether the diseased kidney needs to be removed must be considered.

The management of Wilms' tumour is entering a difficult phase where the results are particularly good and ways of limiting the treatment, particularly the chemotherapy, are being looked at. This is a dangerous phase in which it is perhaps tempting to limit the treatment too far. There has been a similar exercise in the management of the rhabdomyosarcoma.

With the increasing use of CT scanning, lung metastases are now seen in some cases of Stage 1 disease that have a negative chest X-ray film. These may be the cases that will not be successful on the simple management of Stage 1 disease already described.

All patients with unfavourable histology are treated with triple chemo-therapy. Furthermore, with unfavourable histology, the decision to give radiotherapy is based on a "second look" laparotomy. Thus, the management of a patient with unfavourable histology is to give triple chemotherapy and then perform a further laparotomy at three months. If there is residual disease, radiotherapy is used. However, the second laparotomy is not universally popular and it may be that it will be abandoned before too long.

There are some conditions which are associated with Wilms' disease such as the Beckwith-Wiederman syndrome. Children with this syndrome (exomphalos, macroglossia and gigantism) are seen every 3 months for the first 2 years and are investigated with ultrasound every 6 months. Over the age of 3 years, they are seen every 6 months and an ultrasound examination is done each year. This approach is perhaps a little illogical, because most of the children who develop a tumour with the Beckwith-Wiederman syndrome present with a mass, but a recent study from the USA has confirmed the safety of the approach in high-risk groups. The risk of Wilms' tumour is not mentioned to the patients or to the parents.

It is reasonable to do a needle biopsy percutaneously in a child with a Stage 4 renal tumour in order to obtain an adequate histology.

In the Manchester series bilateral renal tumours were found in one in a series of 50 cases, but in other series there is a 5%–10% rate. The problem of nephroblastomatosis makes it extremely difficult to decide whether one is really dealing with a Wilms' tumour and this makes the diagnosis of bilateral Wilms' tumour particularly difficult.

Testicular Tumours

Manchester is either the second or third largest paediatric oncology unit in the UK and only three testicular tumours have been seen there in 7 years: these are all orchioblastomas or teratomas. Leydig tumours are rarer and produce androgenic effects in late childhood with precocious puberty. Other tumours include seminoma, gonadoblastoma and paratesticular tumours or rhabdomyosarcoma. Secondary tumours include the leukaemic children who get deposits of tumour within the testicle. Thus, the vast majority of testicular tumours will be teratomas or orchioblastomas (Table 4.5).

Teratomas and orchioblastomas are usually seen in young children from around the age of 2 years. The teratoma grows slowly and the orchioblastoma grows quickly, and both present as an enlarged testis which does not transilluminate. Provided that this is borne in mind they will not be mistaken for a hydrocele. Teratomas are mostly benign. There has been discussion as to whether these should be shelled out, but the whole testis is replaced by tumour and there is no question of anything other than an orchidectomy. Patients with orchioblastoma show increased levels in alphafetoprotein (AFP) and sometimes HCG. These levels must be estimated before removal of the testis. If the levels of these markers return to normal within a month, no further treatment is necessary. If they remain high, this is an indication that there is spread of tumour and chemotherapy is then given for 6 months. All such patients on the Manchester Tumour Registry have survived. The teratomas need simple orchidectomy and no further treatment as they are nearly always benign. It is probably worth noting that the AFP is normally raised for a few months after birth and this can lead to confusion in the presence of a testicular mass; these tumours usually present after this initial neonatal period so confusion is not likely.

Table 4.5. Testis tumours in children

Orchioblastoma	55% (Raised AFP/HCG)
Teratoma	35% (Occasionally, raised AFP/HCG)
Leydig tumour	Rare (Androgenic effects)
Seminoma	Rare
Gonadoblastoma	Rare
Paratesticular rhabdomyosarcoma	Rare
Secondary tumour from leukaemia	Rare

Further Reading

Gilchrist GS, Kelalis PP (1976) Tumors and related disorders. In: Kelalis PP, King LR (eds) Clinical pediatric urology, Chapter 25. Saunders, Philadelphia

Dialogues in pediatric urology (1984) Rhabdomyosarcoma of bladder, prostate and vagina. Vol 7, No 4
Dialogues in pediatric urology (1984) Yolk sac tumors: current management Vol 7, No 11
Dialogues in pediatric urology (1985) Bilateral Wilms' tumour. Vol 8, No 10
Dialogues in pediatric urology (1988) Wilms' tumor update: current issues in management. Vol 11, No 11

Chapter 5

Prenatal Diagnosis

David F. M. Thomas and Robert H. Whitaker

Prenatal diagnosis is revolutionising paediatric urology, and will alter both the practice and also the understanding of many of the abnormalities. One of the effects of this will be a move in emphasis towards the practice of paediatric urology. Since so many of the conditions that otherwise might have presented later in childhood or even in adulthood will now be diagnosed prenatally, decisions will have to be made and surgical treatment undertaken in the neonatal period or in early infancy by those who are practised in operating on small children. The accuracy of ultrasound imaging has improved immeasurably over the last decade. It now provides very fine detail down to a resolution of a millimetre or less and by screening the mother in pregnancy one can pick up many abnormalities of the fetus. Collections of fluid show up particularly well with ultrasound. It is not surprising, therefore, that conditions such as hydronephrosis and dilatation of the cerebral ventricles are particularly well seen. Soft tissue abnormalities such as exomphalos and other mid-line defects can also be detected. Diaphragmatic hernias can also be seen together with other gut abnormalities and it is possible to diagnose many of the congenital cardiac anomalies in utero.

Abnormalities of the urinary tract are amongst those that are looked for routinely in most major obstetric centres, but we are still heavily dependant upon the skill and expertise of the person who is performing the ultrasound examination. Between 17 and 19 weeks of gestation ultrasound imaging can see 95% of fetal kidneys; hydronephrosis can be seen even earlier than 17 weeks. Sometimes the images are extremely difficult to interpret, but they are getting easier as the definition of imaging improves. One of the problems is distinguishing the normal from the abnormal. For example, a renal pelvis of 6-mm diameter is probably just within the normal limits although, with increasing experience, a renal pelvis of up to 1-cm diameter is probably acceptable.

Nowadays it should be possible to diagnose a hydronephrosis and a multicystic kidney with considerable ease.

How common are these abnormalities? In the population in Leeds nearly 95% of all pregnancies are scanned. The scans are not always performed at times when it is possible to guarantee to pick up all the abnormalities since many studies are performed in the very early stages of pregnancy. In the 4 years to the end of 1986 over 90% of 37 000 births were scanned and 45 major uropathies were detected, representing significant abnormalities in 1 in 800 live births. The incidence of congenital renal anomalies reported in large autopsy studies is of the order of 1 in 500 to 1 in 1000. For example, the study of 245 000 autopsies reported by Ashley and Mostofi (1960) quoted a figure of 1 in 650. The pick-up rate for antenatal ultrasound of 1 in 800 suggests that the majority of renal anomalies are now being detected before birth. The pick-up rate is not as high in district hospitals, but in time it will be: soon, it will be possible to pick up all significant renal abnormalities.

Some of the earlier figures may help to answer some questions about the value of prenatal diagnosis. In the 4 years up to 1986 there were 105 fetuses in whom abnormalities were detected. They were referred in utero or promptly in the postnatal period. Of the 105, 7 were thought to have sufficiently gross abnormality with oligohydramnios and gross renal dysplasia that the pregnancy should be terminated and, in every instance, the histology confirmed that these were grossly dysplastic kidneys. Of 98 live-born neonates, 23 had mild transient dilatation and 75 had what proved to be a significant degree of uropathy; the distribution of bilateral and unilateral pathology is shown in Fig. 5.1.

In some instances one could argue that prenatal diagnosis of the renal abnormality was irrelevant. For instance, prenatal diagnosis was not needed to tell one that there is something very wrong with a child born with gross abdominal distension, a Potter's facies and pulmonary hypoplasia. In addition 15 children had clinical signs which would have prompted investigation of the

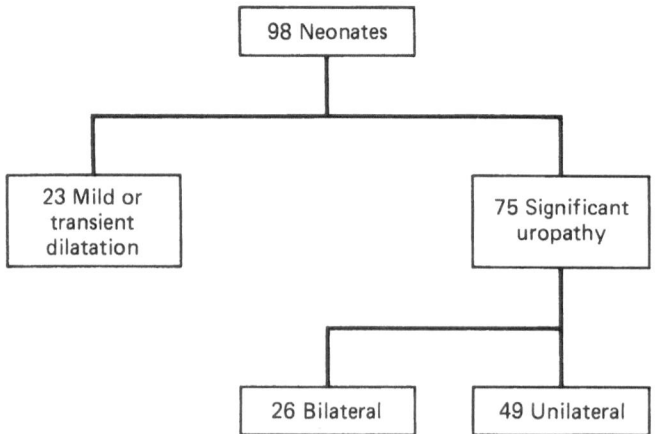

Fig. 5.1. Uropathies found in 98 live-born neonates in whom abnormalities had been detected prenatally.

child immediately after birth in the absence of ultrasound imaging results. Ultrasound, however, alerted the urologist to the need for rapid investigation postnatally but the abnormality would certainly have been found without the prenatal ultrasound. So, in 15 children ultrasound information did not make a lot of difference clinically, but in more than 80% of the cases there were no physical signs and these were problems that would have been missed without ultrasound (Table 5.1). The question is whether it matters if the mildly dilated urinary tracts had been missed: and the answer is that it probably does not.

Table 5.1. The value of ultrasound imaging in the investigation of 98 neonates

Clinical signs present	15 (15.3%)
No clinical signs present	
Ultrasound imaging alone	83
Definite value	16 (16.3%)
Probable value	44 (44.8%)
Doubtful value	23 (23.5%)

Significant Uropathy

There were some cases in which ultrasound was of real value in that the child benefitted from having the urological problem diagnosed prenatally, because more prompt action was possible with, hopefully, a modified prognosis. There was a larger group of children in whom the information was of value in that the abnormality was unilateral but the children would have survived regardless of whether or not the unilateral problem had been detected.

In the "definite value" group, the pathology was treatable and included both bilateral problems and abnormalities of a solitary kidney. The largest single group were infants with a posterior urethral valve. Amongst the bilateral pathology was bilateral pelvi-ureteric obstruction, bilateral reflux or a combination of multicystic kidney on one side and pelvi-ureteric obstruction on the other.

The boys with a posterior urethral valve represent 10% of the significant abnormalities detected. The question here is whether drainage of these high pressure systems in utero can modify the outcome. Of all the uropathies seen in utero this is the only one that is likely to benefit from drainage, although all that may be necessary is to detect these boys in utero so that prompt action can be taken as soon as they are born, by preventing infection. At present the answer about the necessity for prenatal intervention is probably unknown. Fig. 5.2 shows a child with a pelvi-ureteric obstruction on the right and a multicystic kidney on the left. The multicystic kidney was removed, a pyeloplasty was performed and the child is now thriving at 2 years. In contrast with this, another child seen recently with a similar combination of pathology was not detected in utero and presented in chronic renal failure at the age of 2 years. A retrospective view of his growth charts showed that his growth was normal for the first 10 months of life and then started to decline. It is tempting to believe that, had his problem been diagnosed at a very early stage, his renal function could have been preserved and the need for dialysis might have been averted.

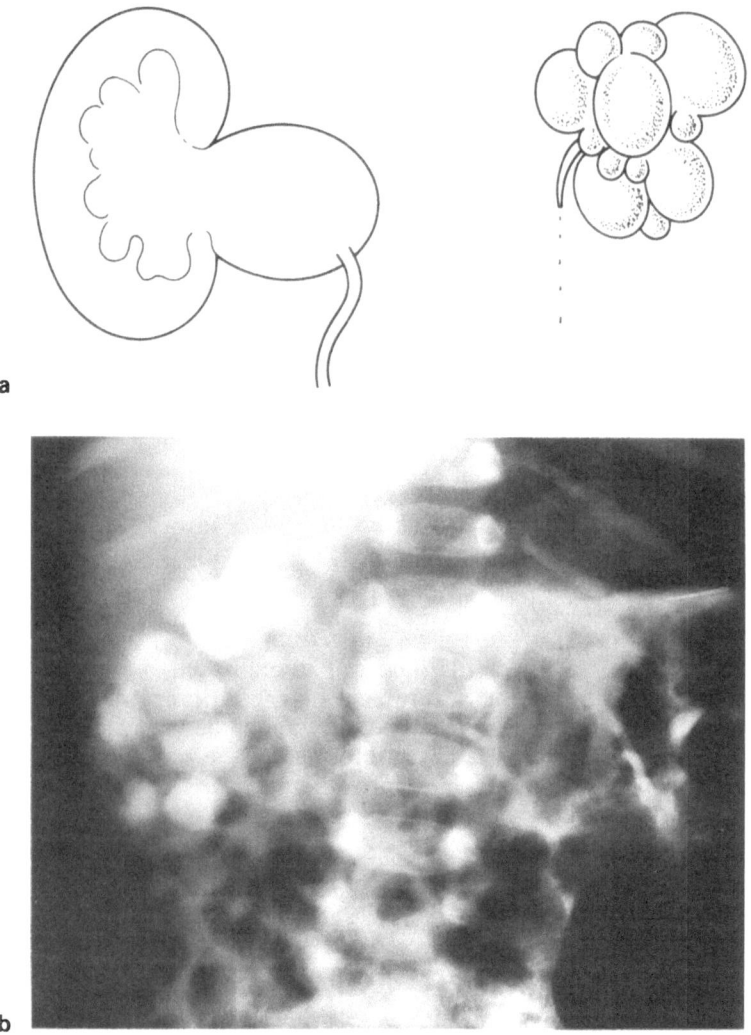

Fig. 5.2a, b. IVU of a child to show a right-sided hydronephrosis due to obstruction of the pelvi-ureteric junction. On the left there is a non-functioning multicystic kidney.

In children with bilateral reflux, it is hoped that, if the reflux is detected in utero and treated with antibiotics from birth, the risk of renal scarring may be minimised. So, there are some children who can undoubtedly be helped by prenatal diagnosis, but they represent a relatively small group of the total number of children.

The biggest single group were children with unilateral significant pathology; pelvi-ureteric obstruction was the largest single group, but other conditions were seen. In this group the information provided by prenatal ultrasound is useful, but not essential. The renal parenchyma is well preserved in the

Table 5.2. Scintigraphic assessment of pelvi-ureteric obstruction

Differential function	Treatment
Greater than 40%	Conservative
10%–40%	Pyeloplasty
Less than 10%	Percutaneous nephrostomy (reassess at 3 weeks)

majority of these children, and the renal pelvis is proportionally much larger than that seen in children presenting at a later age. The renal pelvis seems more compliant in infancy; this may be beneficial in that it takes the pressure off the renal parenchyma. It is now well documented that the IVU is of limited use in the first few weeks of life and, similarly, radionuclide scans can be extremely misleading. For this reason, functional imaging can be deferred until the fourth week of life.

Ransley's scheme for management of these children may be followed and, provided that the renal function is well documented. If there is good preservation of function even in the presence of an obstructed isotope curve, treatment can be deferred (Table 5.2). If function is compromised, a pyeloplasty is needed in the first four to six weeks of life. With very poor renal function, the child is assessed by putting a percutaneous nephrostomy in place and rescanning with DMSA at three weeks. In 4 such patients renal function has been found to have improved to the point where it was felt worthwhile performing a pyeloplasty. There has been considerable debate as to the best time for a pyeloplasty in these children, but in general the tendency is swinging away from very early intervention unless there is evidence of markedly impaired function.

Multicystic Kidney

In multicystic kidneys the parenchyma is replaced by tense cysts and the renal pelvis and upper ureter are usually atretic. Prenatal ultrasound has shown that multicystic kidney is more common than was previously recognised; its incidence is approximately 1 in 4500 live births. Most of these would have gone undiagnosed in the days before prenatal diagnosis. Nowadays with ultrasound and a DMSA scan, one can make the diagnosis with a considerable degree of accuracy. Formerly, these kidneys were removed, and indeed some people still do so, but there is no evidence supporting this action. If the children are followed with ultrasound, regression and disappearance of the cysts can be demonstrated. Many cases of "renal agenesis" started off with a multicystic kidney. The world literature on multicystic kidneys over a 20-year period shows 9 serious complications (hypertension or malignant change). At the moment the onus is on those who recommend early surgery to show that there is a good reason for removing the kidney.

Reflux

Prenatal scanning probably has an important role in the diagnosis of reflux. We have detected 15 examples of reflux prenatally of which 14 were in boys. It is difficult to estimate how many of these would have gone undetected. Of the patients in whom reflux was diagnosed, two subsequently ran into trouble and needed a vesicostomy, but the remainder were managed successfully by conservative treatment; one of these children has now had ureters reimplanted. Because of the technical difficulties of reimplanting refluxing ureters in the neonatal period it is best to defer surgery and either perform a vesicostomy (if necessary) or give continuous antibiotic therapy until the child is older.

Mild Dilatation

There are 23 examples of transient or mild dilatation. For a period micturating cystograms were performed, but they were not rewarding in terms of detecting reflux and they have now been abandoned. The difficult diagnostic dilemma is whether these mildly dilated systems are due to reflux or whether there is a potential for obstruction which may become obvious in later childhood or even in adulthood. One can see, therefore, that there are several unanswered questions in this group.

Fetal Surgery

It is now possible to drain an obstructed urinary tract in utero. The first approach to this was reported from San Francisco and consisted of hysterotomy, delivery of the fetus and open ureterostomies (Harrison et al. 1982). That has now been abandoned in favour of suprapubic shunting with a double J or pigtail catheter to drain the fetal urine into the amniotic fluid. There was great enthusiasm for this some 4 or 5 years ago when it was performed on a largely uncontrolled basis. There is now a world registry for fetal surgery run by Professor Manning in Winnipeg, and the results of 73 cases have been reported (Manning et al. 1986) (Table 5.3). Of the 73 patients, no firm diagnosis was reached in 33. Amongst these there were some examples of the prune belly syndrome and it is doubtful whether they benefitted from drainage. It is likely that only a very small number of these children will benefit from having their urinary tract drained in utero, but the big problem is that we do not yet have the ability to identify those fetuses who would benefit. In the present state of knowledge obstetricians should probably be discouraged from intervening but if they feel strongly that intervention is indicated then, in Great Britain, they should be referred to Kings College Hospital or Queen Charlotte's Hospital for further information. The only possible indication for intervention would be bilateral obstructive uropathy; there is no place for drainage of a unilateral

Table 5.3. The outcome of 73 cases of fetal obstructive uropathy (Fetal Surgery Register 1985)

Diagnosis	No of cases	Total (%)	Survivors (%)
Posterior urethral valve	21	28.8	76.2
Abnormal karyotype	6	8.2	0
Renal dysplasia	5	6.8	0
Urethral atresia	5	6.8	20
Prune belly	3	4.1	100
Unknown aetiology	33	45.3	30.3
Total	73	100	41

hydronephrosis. Other major abnormalities should be excluded since one would not wish to drain the urinary tract of a child with other life-threatening anomalies. In Harrison's group in San Francisco, the most common form of intervention now is termination of pregnancy; the indications for termination are shown in Table 5.4. One would, of course, want to terminate before 24 weeks in view of the current UK Abortion Act, especially if there is severe oligohydramnios due to high grade urinary obstruction in the fetus. On ultrasound these kidneys are often dysplastic and are typically small, bright and echo-dense. Fetal urinary sodium and other urinary constituents should be measured routinely as the inability of the fetal kidney to concentrate urine is the best indicator of severe damage. At the same time a chromosomal analysis is needed. It is likely, therefore, that termination will become the most commonly performed procedure for fetuses with severe urinary abnormalities.

Table 5.4. Criteria for termination

Less than 24 weeks gestation
Oligohydramnios
Small "bright" kidneys
Fetal urinary sodium greater than 100 mmol/l.
Chromosomal or other major defect

Fig. 5.3 shows a scheme for the management of children who are found prenatally to have renal abnormalities. The first question is whether there is dilatation of the ureters. If both ureters are dilated then reflux and/or infra-vesical obstruction must be excluded. If there is any doubt at all a cystogram should be performed in the neonatal period. Outflow obstruction should be treated accordingly. If there is no reflux or outflow obstruction then presumably one is dealing with a lower uretero-vesical obstruction, in which case nothing else is necessary in the immediate neonatal period. If it is certain that there is obstruction at the pelvi-ureteric level, functional imaging should be deferred until 3 or 4 weeks since the information that is given before that time can be very misleading. With a mildly dilated system the question is whether one does a cystogram to look for reflux. A cystogram may be deemed unnecessary: if one is not performed the child is scanned again at 1 month and if the dilatation is still present, the child joins the system described for confirmed dilatation. If there is still mild dilatation or if the system is normal at a month, the child is scanned again at a year and then discharged if this scan is normal. It is possible

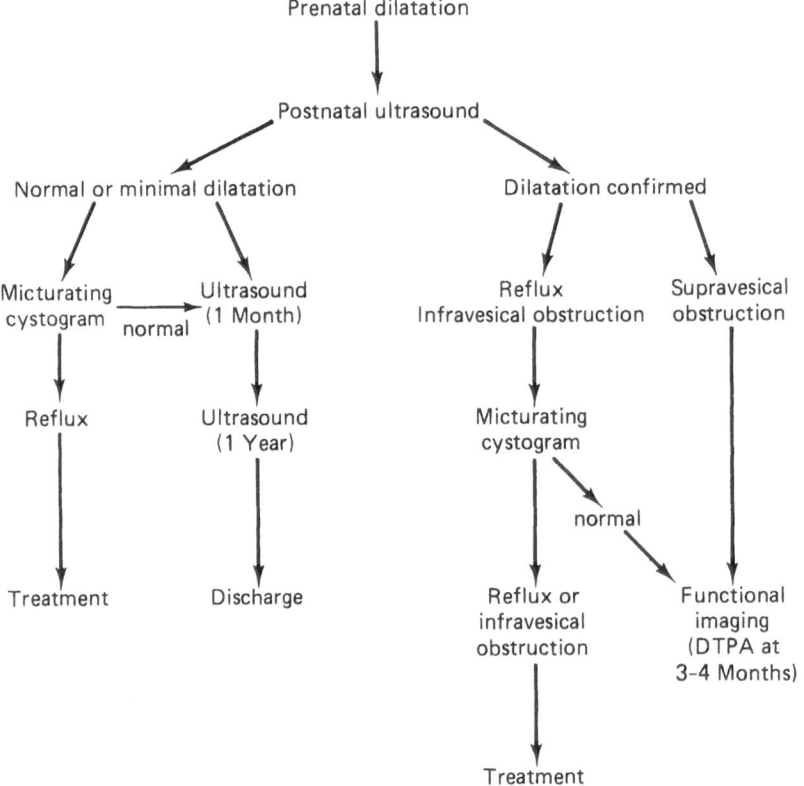

Fig. 5.3. Scheme for the management of children found prenatally to have renal abnormalities.

that some children may be discharged who go on to get trouble in later life but, at the moment, there are insufficient facilities to follow a large number of children on an indefinite basis.

A patient with a pelvi-ureteric junction obstruction diagnosed prenatally and confirmed postnatally can often be left for a year before the obstruction is repaired because the natural history of untreated pelvi-ureteric junction obstruction is not known; for instance, some of these "obstructions" may resolve spontaneously. Pelvi-ureteric obstruction is a relatively benign disease: from a large series of pyeloplasties very good results are seen with a nephrectomy rate of 5% or less in most series. There is no evidence yet to say that these operations must be carried out in the neonatal period.

It has been pointed out (Gough, personal communication) that the studies from Bristol by Roberts and Slade showed that in all the diagnosed cases and in all the post-mortem cases pelvi-ureteric obstruction seemed never to be a benign condition, and that 30 or so patients who had refused operation finally came back asking for it within a 3-year period (Roberts et al. 1972). Two-thirds of the rest of the patients who had been followed showed deterioration by all the various imaging modalities that were available. These were, of course, not antenatal cases but established hydronephrosis in older people. Although one wants to know the natural history, once the diagnosis of obstruction has been established Gough considers that it may not be ethical to do nothing in order to find out what happens if nothing is done.

However, spontaneous resolution of hydronephrosis has been documented in some patients whereas some neonatal pyeloplasties have needed reoperation because of complications. Although Herbert Johnston's series showed that an effective pyeloplasty in the neonatal period was an extremely safe and successful operation, there have been series from respectable centres showing that children who have a pyeloplasty for prenatally diagnosed pelvi-ureteric obstruction may need reoperation and some series contain a very high incidence of complications. It seems that one is aiming for a theoretical marginal increase in the glomerular filtration rate and some kidneys are put at a greater risk purely by operating on them.

It has been pointed out that once a patient has been told that he has a kidney abnormality he is likely to produce symptoms in the next few months. All urologists will have seen many elderly patients with dilated renal pelvis that can be shown to be unobstructed and not giving symptoms; pressure flow studies on a number of elderly patients have nearly always shown that they are not obstructed. In fact, as a general rule, elderly people with equivocal pelvi-ureteric obstruction rarely have significant obstruction. Many neonates undergo growth of the renal pelvis and the pelvi-ureteric junction in such a way that the resistance becomes lower over the months and the obstruction lessens. These are the ones that probably end up as elderly patients with a non-obstructed hydronephrosis. There is good compliance and no functional deterioration.

References

Ashley DJB, Mostofi FK (1960) Renal agenesis and dysgenesis. J Urol 83: 211–230
Harrison MR, Golbus MS, Filly RA et al. (1982) Fetal surgery for congenital hydronephrosis. N Engl J Med 306: 591–593
Manning FA, Harrison MR, Rodeck C et al. (1986) Catheter shunts for fetal hydronephrosis and hydrocephalus. N Engl J Med 315: 336–340
Roberts M, Slade N, Jeffery P (1972) Late results in the management of primary pelvic hydronephrosis. Br J Urol 44: 15–18

Further Reading

Colodny AH (1987) Antenatal diagnosis and management of urinary abnormalities. Pediatr Clin North Am 34: 1365–1381
Crombleholme TM, Harrison MR, Longaker MT, Langer JC (1988) Prenatal diagnosis and management of bilateral hydronephrosis. Pediatr Nephrol 2: 334–342
Gray DL, Crane JP (1988) Prenatal diagnosis of urinary tract malformation. Pediatr Nephrol 2: 326–333
Scott JES, Renwick M (1988) Antenatal diagnosis of congenital abnormalities of the urinary tract. Br J Urol 62: 295–300
Thomas DFM, Irving HC, Arthur RJ (1985) Prenatal diagnosis: how useful is it? Br J Urol 57: 784–787

Chapter 6

The Management of Pelvi-ureteric Junction Obstruction in Neonates

Philip G. Ransley

The most important thing to remember is that there is no indication for any immediate relief of obstruction in the first 24 or 48 hours in any children with pelvi-ureteric junction obstruction. The obstruction has been present for 9 months and did not need any attention during that time so it is best left alone in the immediate postnatal period. After 48 hours a good ultrasound examination can be helpful, but before that time the kidneys may not be producing very much urine and the findings can be misleading. There are many patients in whom the kidney was dilated prenatally, who did not seem to have much dilatation in the first 24 hours of life, and who then became dilated again later. Therefore, there is no need to rush into precipitate surgery.

The question of pelvi-ureteric junction obstruction was first addressed some years ago, when it was recognised, with the advent of prenatal diagnosis, that increasing numbers of these children would be seen. A protocol was established at an early stage from which the natural history of the disease would be learned. As with reflux 25 or 30 years ago, at the outset a conservative programme was followed. Obstruction in the neonate is a very considerable problem; this includes not only pelvi-ureteric obstruction but also posterior urethral valves, ureteroceles and reflux. The diagnosis of these conditions is progressively bringing down the age of the children seen by the paediatric urologist. Recently, there were 22 patients on a 20-bedded ward at Great Ormond Street and not one of them was over 6 months of age. There will be a lot of pressure on paediatric hospitals in the future to cope with all the paediatric urology.

This discussion centres on cases that have a prenatal diagnosis of dilatation which persists postnatally. They have a normal bladder and urethra and the appearances are compatible with pelvi-ureteric obstruction. Some of these children may have reflux, most of them being just a flick of reflux into an undilated ureter, but one or two of them have more severe reflux. We reviewed in October 1987 all our cases from 1980 to the end of 1986. There were 102 kidneys in 80 patients. In 22 patients the problem was judged to be bilateral. The follow-up is at least 1 year for 102 kidneys, 2 years for 67 kidneys, 3 years for 42 kidneys and 31 of them for more than 4 years; we are just beginning to see some early results. Fortunately, hydronephrosis is much more easily defined than a boy with a posterior urethral valve and causes fewer problems in the postnatal period. A prenatally diagnosed hydronephrosis would be followed up with an ultrasound scan during the first week of life. It is probably advisable to avoid a cystogram during the first month of life because of the risk of infection, which at this age can be quite severe. However, in a male child with bilateral hydronephrosis or any child with an abnormal bladder on ultrasound, a micturating cystogram must be done early. In a child with a unilateral hydronephrosis and a normal bladder on ultrasound, the cystogram can be deferred until after the first 3 months of life. Having made a diagnosis of an isolated upper tract problem from the first ultrasound, renal imaging can be deferred until 1 month of age in all children. The reason for this is to allow the rapidly maturing nephrons to develop. The GFR is increasing very rapidly during the first month after which it slows. At 1 month one can get reasonable base-line information. In the early part of the study cases were assessed and treatment decided on the basis of the scan at 1 month. In recent years the only patients subjected to intervention were those with very poorly functioning kidneys; the remainder were left until 3 months, at which time a management decision was made on the basis of a 3-month DTPA scan. They were then classified into three entirely arbitrary groups based on proportional function: (1) fewer than 20% are defined as poor (the DTPA scan probably cannot differentiate between 5% and 20%), (2) moderate (20%–40%) and (3) good function (over 40%). In the presence of bilateral hydronephrosis the problem is much more difficult and it then becomes a matter of judgement based on the computer analysis and the analogue images to classify the individual kidneys appropriately. This is a weakness in the study but there is no alternative to it at the moment. The groupings are so crude that this error does not matter.

In 102 kidneys, 8 fell into the very poor function group, 24 into the moderate function group, and 70 into the group defined as good function with unilateral dilatation (Table 6.1). At 1 month, the patients in the poor function group had a pigtail catheter put into the kidney percutaneously. At 3 months, the moderate

Table 6.1. Treatment of 102 kidneys, with a prenatal diagnosis of dilatation that persists postnatally

		Surgery	Conservative treatment
Poor (8)	Nephrectomy	4	
	Pyeloplasty	4	
Moderate (24)	Pyeloplasty	20	4
Good (70)	Pyeloplasty		
	Early	4	54
	Late	12	

group underwent a pyeloplasty. The good group had further scans at 6 months, 1 year and 2 years, and beyond that as necessary. They were all put on antibiotics, usually Trimethoprim alone in a dose of 1 to 2 mg/kg per day. At the moment the policy is slightly arbitrary in that antibiotics are maintained until one year, and are then discontinued.

Poor Function Group

In the poor function group there was a 50/50 split between pyeloplasty and nephrectomy after pigtail drainage (Table 6.1). Fig. 6.1 shows one of the good children in this poor group—hydronephrosis on ultrasound imaging and a DTPA scan showing a very poor functioning kidney on the left. A second DTPA scan was performed after 5 weeks of pigtail drainage and a further scan at 9 months after a pyeloplasty. In this classification of function the uptake component of the curve only is considered. No notice is taken of post-lasix drainage curves since it is function that is of interest and not drainage.

Moderate Function Group

In the moderate function group there were 24 kidneys (Table 6.2), and 20 had a pyeloplasty. The classification of "improved ++" means that function came back to the same as the opposite side. They are "improved +" if function increases but does not return to the same as the opposite side. There was no change in 9 kidneys and one was lost to follow-up. Thus, 9 out of 20 showed no change with moderately depressed function after a pyeloplasty at 1–3 months; 5 showed good improvement and 5 showed some improvement. Some children disappeared from immediate follow-up and this group, therefore, had no treatment: 3 of 4 such children spontaneously "improved ++" to equal function with the opposite side. These are better results statistically than those in the pyeloplasty group although the numbers are small. The question arises as to whether the function really is recoverable or whether there was obstruction at all. If the concept of transient outflow obstruction is a valid one, there may also be a similar transient type of obstruction at the pelvi-ureteric junction. There may, therefore, be two separate groups—one group representing residual hydronephrosis after a burnt-out prenatal obstruction, and the other a

Table 6.2. Group with moderate function (24 kidneys)

		No. of kidneys
Pyeloplasty (20)	Improved ++	5
	Improved +	5
	No change	9
	No follow-up	1
Conservative (4)	Improved	3
	No change	1

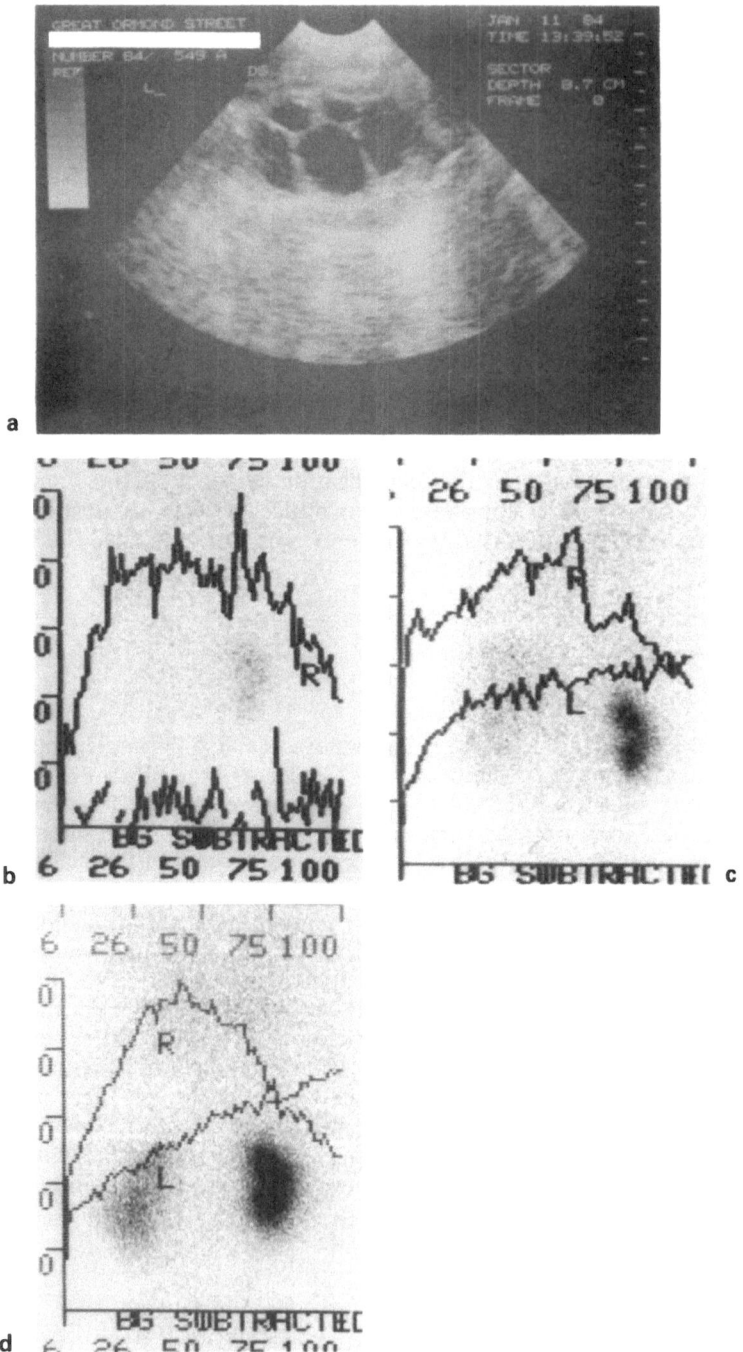

Fig. 6.1a, b, c, d.   Example of a child in the poor group in whom adequate renal function was obtained with appropriate treatment. Ultrasound, **a**, and DTPA, **b**, showing poor function on the left. Repeat DTPA, **c**, after 5 weeks of pigtail treatment, showing improved function. DTPA, **d**, 9 months after a left pyeloplasty, showing maintained improved function.

true obstructive hydronephrosis. It will be interesting to sort this out in years to come. In summary, half the children who showed moderately reduced function improved their function after pyeloplasty.

Good Function Group

The good function group is the largest and therefore, of course, the most important. Table 6.1 shows that 4 of these had an early pyeloplasty. These may be dismissed as they are no longer of any interest. There is at least a 1-year follow-up on all 66 cases that were followed conservatively, 2–3 years on 41, more than 3 years on 22 and more than 4 years on 16. In the first year of follow-up, 7 out of the 66 underwent a pyeloplasty simply because they were thought to need one; in the second year, 4 out of 41 needed a pyeloplasty and, in the third year, 1 out of 22. In the 16 cases that have been followed for between 4 and 7 years there has been no indication for a pyeloplasty. Thus, 12 out of the 66 came to pyeloplasty because they developed a problem in the postnatal period. A strict protocol was followed to avoid bias in the results, but at times this was found difficult. The difficulty is illustrated by a child who had an IVU after transfer from another hospital with a palpable kidney following an antenatal diagnosis. The kidney shows "soap bubbles" and the delayed film shows the classical ground-glass appearance of a severe hydronephrosis. The initial DTPA study at 1 month was satisfactory, so he had no intervention. At 6 months the DTPA suggested that there was less function on that side so we did an antegrade pyelogram which confirmed the diagnosis of pelvi-ureteric obstruction. He was restudied 3 months after a pyeloplasty and there was considerable improvement in function. This case illustrates, yet again, that there is probably no great urgency in surgical management.

If, then, the 12 patients who had pyeloplasty are analysed it is seen that 7 of them were operated upon for reduced function. Of these, 3 returned to their original levels, 1 showed some improvement and 3 recent cases have not yet had their follow-up studies. A urinary tract infection for which a pyeloplasty was performed developed in 2 cases, and 1 child developed pain. Another child developed a severe concentrating defect and polyuria and one had surgery for increasing parenchymal transit time on a scintiscan, an investigation we used in the early stages. It can be seen that the commonest cause for intervention is deteriorating renal function.

Thus, out of the 102 kidneys there have been 4 nephrectomies, 4 inappropriate early pyeloplasties in the good group, 4 good pyeloplasties in the poor functioning group and 32 pyeloplasties that may or may not have been necessary in other groups. Perhaps more important are the 58 kidneys that are getting on very well indeed without any intervention. This type of study is needed to put our practice on a firm footing.

There have been no major problems with infections developing in this study. The children have been on prophylactic antibiotics. One of the infections was extremely doubtful in a child from a medical family. The child was unwell with a mild fever. Another one was unwell for a very short time. If the children were acutely ill they would be referred straight back to us and if they were very sick a percutaneous pigtail catheter would be inserted without hesitation to drain the kidney.

The radiation dose to the kidneys from repeated isotope studies is a slight worry, but in fact all the scans in the first year of life add up to less than one IVU. The biggest worry, if there is an obstruction, is that the isotope is not cleared adequately from the kidney.

The need is now to refine the programme; there is no vested interest in not operating on these children. If at the end of the day it is shown that every single one of the patients ends up needing a pyeloplasty, then the conclusion must be that here is a problem that is not urgent, that it does eventually lead to trouble and a planned pyeloplasty can be carried out at about 6 months. But there must be proof that this approach is necessary: if 50% of the children get better and never need an operation, a selective mechanism will be retained. Fewer scans will be needed in future than are used now.

Lowell King is a great supporter of early pyeloplasty in the neonatal period. He makes the point that the upper ureter is dilated below the pelvi-ureteric junction in these very young children and that the pyeloplasty at this stage is much easier than later on. However this, by itself, is not a good enough reason for operating.

Further Reading

Dialogues in Pediatric Urology (1987) Renal physiology and obstructive uropathy in the fetus and newborn. Vol.10, No 7

Dialogues in Pediatric Urology (1988) Ureteropelvic junction obstruction in neonates: Renal scanning's role. Vol.11, No 10

Gonzales ET (1985) Genitourinary disorders in the neonate. In: Whitaker RH, Woodward JR (eds) Pediatric urology. Butterworths, London, pp. 167–227

Chapter 7

Equivocal Upper Tract Obstruction

Robert H. Whitaker

It is difficult to summarise what we have covered so far in this volume on the topic of obstruction, but it is admirable that Philip Ransley has decided that the main diagnostic criterion should be renal function. It seems that he is including amongst his cases for conservative management ones which are obstructed, but which still retain moderately good function, in whom the obstruction either gets worse or better. Many of the cases which improve are examples of fetal folds—those convoluted upper ureters that were seen so often on urograms in neonates. They are not always demonstrable on the intravenous urogram but can be seen on an antegrade pyelogram during perfusion, but several cases have been found where fetal folds have disappeared. There are also some cases at the age of 5 or 6 years that still have these fetal folds, and pressure measurements in these children have shown that there is a true obstruction.

First, it is necessary to consider the radiographic signs of obstruction that urologists tend to rely on: the only true sign of obstruction during an IVU is extravasation of contrast medium. All other factors in Table 7.1 are less reliable and become more so as one passes down the list ending up with general dilatation which is, of course, not necessarily synonymous with obstruction.

Table 7.1. Radiological signs of obstruction arranged in order of reliability

1. Extravasation
2. Excessively delayed drainage
3. Persistent nephrogram
4. Negative pyelogram
5. Poor ureteric filling
6. Caliceal change
7. General dilatation

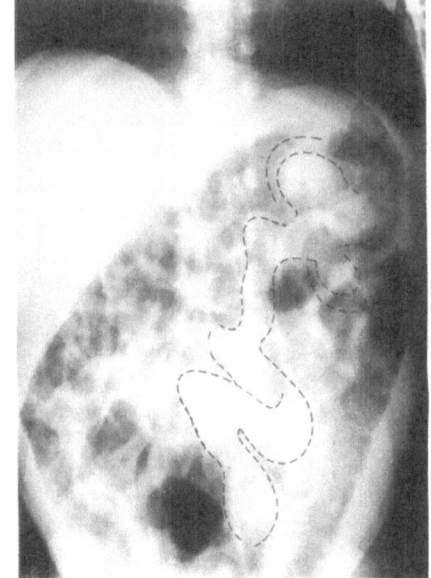

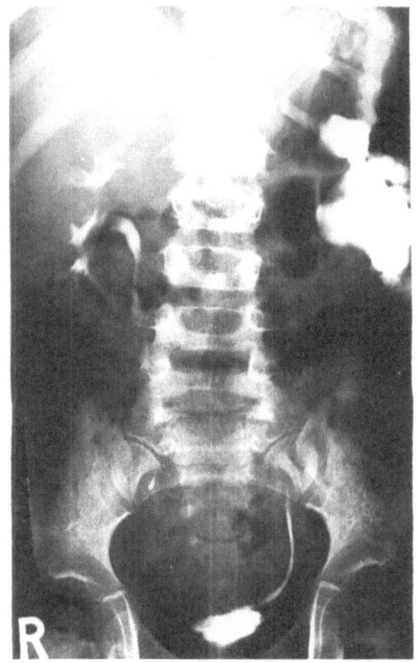

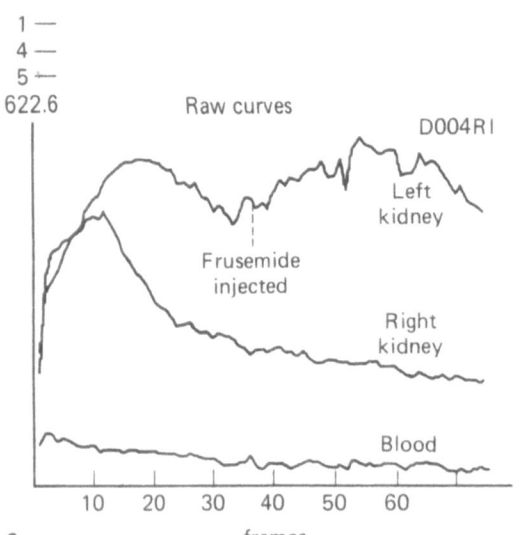

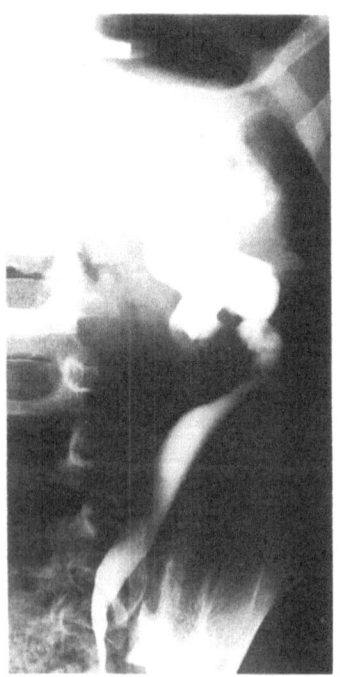

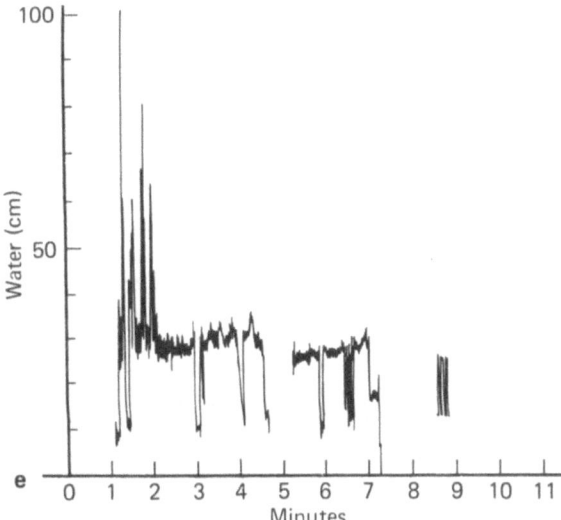

Fig. 7.1a, b, c, d, e. Child with an obstructed left megaureter **a**, Initial IVU; the interrupted line shows the outline of the megaureter; **b**, IVU after restoration of continuity, suggesting a left hydronephrosis; **c**, renogram suggesting obstruction; **d**, pressure flow study showing free drainage with no obstruction, but odd configuration because of previous ureterostomy; **e**, pressure flow tracing showing no obstruction.

It is clear that in the prune belly syndrome there is considerable dilatation without obstruction. The caliceal changes are often unimportant. For instance, in megacalicosis there is no obstruction. Poor ureteric filling clearly cannot be so important. For many years it was believed that if the ureter was not seen to fill well on the static X-ray film of an IVU it was obstructed, but this cannot be the case in a functioning kidney. A negative pyelogram is unreliable because it can still be seen after the relief of obstruction and a persistent nephrogram can be seen in any patient whose blood pressure lowers as may occur during an adverse reaction to contrast. Thus, any one of these signs is probably unreliable by itself. A combination of several of them becomes more meaningful.

Fig. 7.1 summarises a case in which a high ureterostomy was performed for a child with a severely obstructed left megaureter (Fig. 7.1a) in the neonatal period. The ureter drained satisfactorily and came back down to a much more normal size. At approximately 6 months a reimplantation of the ureter was performed and the ureterostomy was closed. A subsequent intravenous urogram suggested (Fig. 7.1b) that there might be an element of pelvi-ureteric obstruction and a renogram was performed (Fig. 7.1c). This suggested a moderately severe degree of obstruction probably at the pelvi-ureteric level, and an antegrade pyelogram was performed with pressure flow studies (Fig. 7.1d, e). This showed that there was perfectly good drainage with a 3–4 cm of water pressure gradient between kidney and bladder, completely excluding obstruction. This is just one of many cases in which the pressure study and the renogram gave diametrically opposite opinions as to the presence or absence of obstruction.

In 32 cases, the renogram and the pressure flow study were compared (Whitaker and Buxton-Thomas 1984). The renogram was performed in the morning and the pressure flow study in the afternoon. If there was a spontaneously falling curve, lasix was not given. If there was a rising curve then lasix was always given. In 12 patients the studies agreed that there was no obstruction, and in 5 they agreed that there was an obstruction. There were 5 where the pressure flow study showed no obstruction, but the renogram showed definite obstruction and 6 vice versa. The equivocal ones can be omitted because if an equivocal result is obtained in any study, a further or alternative study is performed to try and clarify the situation. If one looks more carefully at the studies which showed evidence of obstruction on the renogram, but where the obstruction was not confirmed on the pressure flow studies (false-positive renograms), there were two consistent features. First, the renal pelvis or the system in general was grossly dilated, and second, the effective renal plasma flow index (ERPFI) was lowered in virtually all these cases, but not to any enormous extent. The amount of renal deterioration necessary before the renogram begins to give unreliable results is, at present, unknown.

The false-negative renograms present even more difficult analysis. These are ones in which the renogram curve appears to be unobstructed yet the pressure flow study shows that there is a definite obstruction. Fig. 7.2 shows a patient with a solitary left kidney with an unobstructed renographic curve (a) and yet the pressure flow study showed a very considerably raised pressure (b). When there is a full diuretic load on a solitary kidney the renogram just simply cannot detect the rise in pressure that is necessary to push the isotope through. Amongst this group there are probably examples of intermittent obstruction. There are times when the pressure flow study will reveal an intermittent obstruction when the renogram will not. Indeed, there are patients in whom nothing can show the intermittent obstruction, short of an IVU during an attack of pain. There is one other patient in this group of false-negative renograms

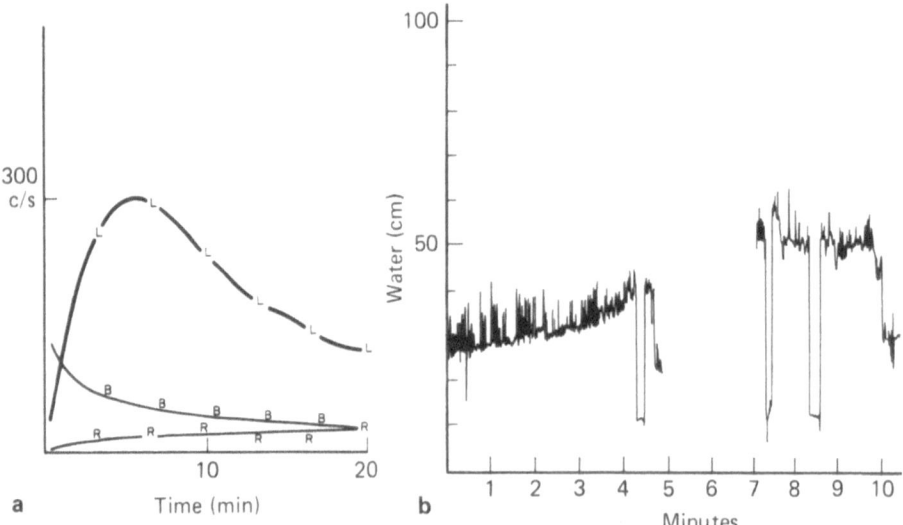

Fig. 7.2a, b. Example of a DTPA showing normal transit (a) but a pressure flow study on this patient (b) showed a high pressure consistent with obstruction.

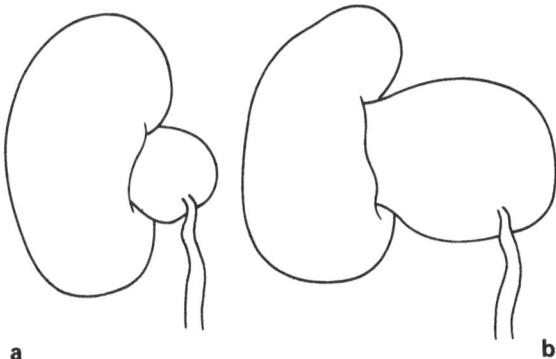

a   b

Fig. 7.3a, b. Compliance is probably very important. A patient, **a**, with a small renal pelvis must reach a maximal volume, and hence danger pressure, faster than a patient with a large renal pelvis, **b**, for a given degree of obstruction and fluid loading.

who had bilateral thin ureters and this can be treated as a similar situation to having a solitary kidney where the total diuretic pressure is equal on both sides. This patient showed consistent evidence of obstruction on repeated pressure flow studies. Thus, in a third of cases the studies do not agree although every urologist must, of course, judge for himself which to believe.

There are three further points that need discussion. One is compliance which is probably important (Bullock and Whitaker 1984). If, for instance, one considers two patients with a relatively small degree of pelvi-ureteric obstruction and one patient has a large renal pelvis whilst the other has a small one they respond in different ways to a fluid load (Fig. 7.3). If these two patients consume a moderate amount of fluid, the patient with the small renal pelvis (a) will soon raise the pressure within it and may very soon reach a danger limit in terms of pressure; the patient with a large renal pelvis but with the same degree of obstruction (b) can consume very much more fluid before the pressure reaches the same danger point. This difference in ability to consume fluid according to the degree of compliance must be taken into account when assessing a patient.

The next point is a question of an increasing flow rate with or without occlusive peristalsis. In 2 patients with equal degrees of uretero-vesical obstruction, one with peristaltic occlusion and one without, it can be seen that at low flow rates the renal pelvic pressure in both is low (Fig. 7.4a, b). When each of these patients is stressed with a diuresis the flow increases and the patient with occlusive peristalsis will raise the pressure within each bolus along the ureter, but the renal pelvic pressure remains low (Fig. 7.4c). The patient with the wide ureter will raise the pressure within the whole system and the pressure will be transmitted back to the kidney and hence to the distal tubules and will prevent them from concentrating adequately (Fig. 7.4d). This, in turn, will cause a further diuresis which will elevate the pressure higher and damage the tubules even more.

Finally, there is the question of why some kidneys show deterioration in renal function over the years. This can be explained to some extent by the fact that, as a child grows, urine production by the kidney will naturally increase and, for a fixed amount of resistance, will cause an increase in pressure; this

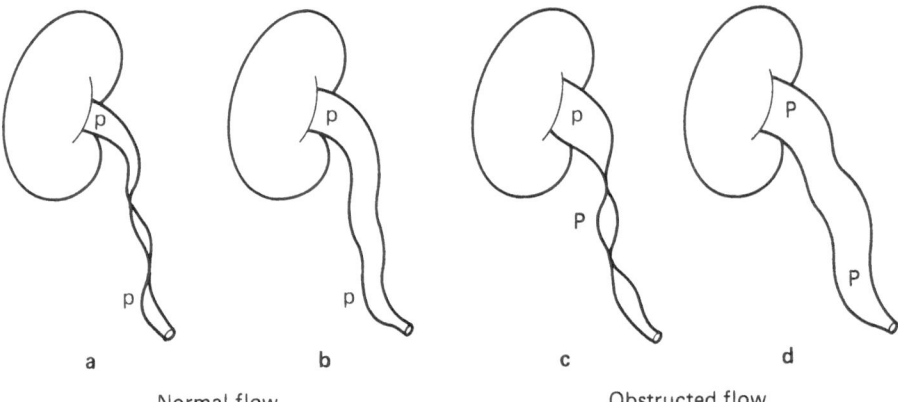

Normal flow   Obstructed flow

Fig. 7.4a, b, c, d.   Occlusive versus non-occlusive peristalsis. See the text for explanation.

may, in turn, cause a deterioration in renal function. Thus, some of the deteriorating kidneys under discussion may be accountable on this basis.

In some cases, at 1 month, looking for objective evidence of obstruction as judged by the third part of the renogram, no objective evidence of obstruction is found. The vast majority of cases, however, have a horizontal or gently rising third phase after lasix. It is important to look at the analogue curve to make sure that the child has emptied the bladder. A full bladder can undoubtedly affect the renal pelvic drainage, and Ransley believes that the most important catheter after a pyeloplasty is the bladder catheter. He suggests that a tubeless pyeloplasty with a bladder catheter is the ideal situation.

These renographic findings are very similar to those of Eric Lupton in Manchester in patients with apparent pelvi-ureteric obstruction whom he has chosen to follow conservatively. He agrees with the natural history study of Roberts and Slade (1964); he found that there is a continuing deterioration in function, but it is a very slow process. There is a need for some objective criteria of obstruction either on a renographic curve or on the basis of a pressure flow study.

It is important to decide at an early stage whether there is any objective evidence of obstruction and to separate the two groups as soon as possible. Philip Ransley has elected not to try to assess the degree of obstruction and that is the basis of his protocol. It is a shame that we do not combine series so that we can measure obstruction by pressure flow studies in all these children to correlate them with the functional changes. It has been shown that there is no slow deterioration after a successful pyeloplasty. The function does not necessarily improve, but at least there is no further deterioration.

The neonatal kidney probably cannot withstand such high pressures as perhaps an older kidney can. Over the years, criteria for obstruction have not been modified but what is done with the knowledge has changed. It is now appreciated that there are older patients with compliant systems that take a long time to fill up whom one is prepared to leave with an element of obstruction. In a series of children who have slightly raised pressures of around about 20–24 cm of water at 10 ml/min progress is simply being watched. Often they are observed because it is not clear what should be done surgically.

As far as the timing of lasix is concerned, it is worth reviewing the papers that have appeared in the literature in the last 2 years; all are aimed at improving the interpretation of the diuretic renogram. The fact that there have been so many papers may suggest that many people find renography imperfect in this situation. Attempts to quantify the renogram with isotope "half lives" are difficult to accept. It is all an effort to make a scientific attribution to something which is totally unscientific and unquantifiable. The only thing that is quantifiable is what Philip Ransley is measuring and that is the ability of the kidney to take in the isotope as it comes through. Beyond that point mixing, peristalsis and all the other factors make the rest of the renographic curve totally unquantifiable. The only people who are entitled to comment on the value of any particular test are those who are comparing it with another one. All too often a test is performed and an operation is done at a later date; with the kidney in the hand the surgeon says "yes, there is the obstruction". This is the way he correlates the study with the operative findings in a most unscientific way; he then looks back and says the test was either right or wrong. Such reports in the literature really do more harm than good. Those people who believe that the renogram is the answer to the diagnosis of obstruction should heed my series which showed in 30% of cases the renogram gave exactly the opposite answer to the pressure flow study.

Although one could be accused of perfusing a kidney unphysiologically at 10 ml/min in a small child, it is known that patients sitting in the ward drinking with a nephrosotomy tube in place have managed to produce a flow rate of 15–18 ml/min/kidney suggesting that this is not grossly unphysiological. It must be remembered that potential obstruction as much as actual obstruction is being searched for.

Even in small children, flow rates of 10 ml/min are maintained because many children without obstruction can tolerate this type of flow without a rise in pressure. If an obstructed curve is observed at 10 ml/min in a small child, the flow is turned down to 5 ml/min; a child is yet to be found who is not still obstructed at 5 ml/min but who was obstructed at 10 ml/min.

The analogy with lower tract urodynamics is worth considering at this point. An enormous amount of information came out of the early studies both from San Francisco and from the Middlesex Hospital that, at the end of the day, could be correlated with the symptoms that emerged from good history taking, and with certain signs on urograms. We have looked back at all the urograms over the years and there are certain features that can be correlated between the pressure flow studies and the urograms. Thus, from looking at a urogram, a very good idea can be gained as to whether or not it is obstructed. If one sees on a post-micturition film an occlusive area within the ureter then one can be really sure that this is not an obstructed system. This is particularly useful in the post-reimplanted ureter. Another feature is a flat edge to the renal pelvis as it lies against the psoas muscle. This tells you that you are dealing with a distensible system but that it is not obstructed at the time of this X-ray examination. However, one must be wary because if there is a full system from top to bottom it does not necessarily mean that it is obstructed. However, if in doubt one would, of course, do a pressure flow study.

Returning for a moment to the criteria for operating on an infant hydro-nephrosis, there is certainly a need to assess function and the patients should be allocated into categories according to function. One must do a percutaneous drainage procedure on the low function group, but one would also perform an antegrade pressure flow study on the group with moderately depressed renal function to make an assessment of obstruction. If they are not obstructed, they should be left, but if they are obstructed they should be operated on.

The approach to preserving or removing a poorly functioning kidney is to some extent a matter of philosophy. One must be prepared to watch carefully in all groups and at the slightest sign of renal deterioration to take appropriate action. One might criticise this approach by saying that some nephrons have been actively destroyed during this waiting period although what one is doing at present would probably avoid most of those problems. My philosophy has always been that we should see if we can predict either whether an obstruction is there now, or whether there is potential for an obstruction that might cause renal function to deteriorate in 5 years' time. From our long-term follow-up study of between 5 and 10 years of 63 cases, mostly from Great Ormond Street, we are happy with the long-term predictive values of the pressure flow studies (Witherow and Whitaker 1981; Wolk and Whitaker 1982).

References

Bullock KN, Whitaker RH (1984) Does good upper tract compliance preserve renal function? J Urol 131: 914–916

Roberts JBM, Slade N (1964) The natural history of primary pelvic hydronephrosis. Br J Surg 51: 759–762

Whitaker RH, Buxton-Thomas M (1984) A comparison of pressure flow studies and renography in equivocal upper urinary tract obstruction. J Urol 131: 446–449

Witherow RO'N, Whitaker RH (1981) The predictive accuracy of antegrade pressure flow studies in equivocal upper tract obstruction. Br J Urol 53: 496–499

Wolk FN, Whitaker RH (1982) Late follow up of dynamic evaluation of upper urinary tract obstruction. J Urol 128: 346–347

Further Reading

Koff SA, Whitaker RH (1985) Recent advances in the diagnosis of upper urinary tract obstruction. In: Whitaker RH, Woodward JR (eds) Pediatric urology. Butterworths, London, pp. 154–166

O'Reilly PH, Gosling JA (eds) (1982) Idiopathic hydronephrosis. Springer-Verlag, Heidelberg

Whitaker RH (1979) The Whitaker test. Urol Clin North Am 6: 529–539

Chapter 8

Urinary Tract Trauma

David C. S. Gough

Major Versus Minor Renal Injury

For every 100 cases of renal contusion there will be a further 7 with renal laceration, 3 with a ruptured kidney, and 3 with a renal vascular pedicle injury, so the chances of any one surgeon seeing very many of these is quite small (Fig. 8.1). The kidney is the commonest single organ that is damaged and is more commonly injured than the spleen. Following in decreasing order of frequency are injuries to the kidney and spleen together, the liver on its own, the liver and spleen and a combination of kidney and liver. Thus, renal injuries in isolation are common. The injury is usually a contusion in which the renal capsule remains intact so there is very little in the way of long-term problems. If there is laceration of the kidney the capsule is usually torn and there is extravasation of blood and sometimes of urine. Complete rupture of the kidney in which there is total disruption of the renal capsule, often with areas of dead kidney, is again a rare lesion. I have only ever seen one pedicle injury. A further, even rarer, type of injury is disruption of the pelvi-ureteric junction unassociated with any other injury. I have never seen such a case.

Contusion

Renal contusion should always be investigated because some 10% of patients have an underlying abnormality which makes the kidney more prone to traumatisation. This is usually a pelvi-ureteric junction obstruction, but can be

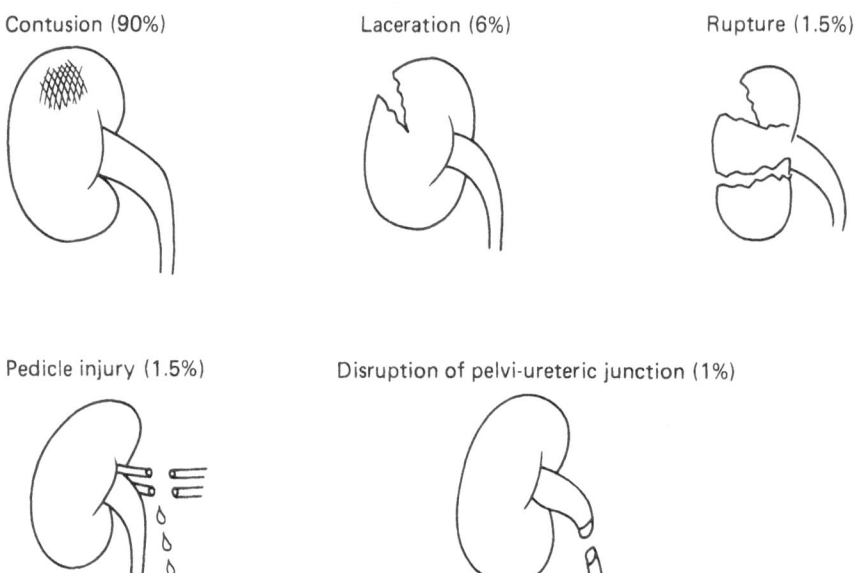

Fig. 8.1. Renal injuries.

vesico-ureteric reflux, a tumour or a horseshoe kidney. All these children should be investigated. From a practical point of view the IVU is still the most useful investigation and it is universally available even in the middle of the night. Ultrasound may also be useful but is more difficult to obtain out-of-hours and can be difficult to perform in the Accident Department on a patient with multiple injuries. A plain X-ray and IVU not only give information about the problem under consideration, but also give information about the prognosis; there is much historical evidence which supports this hypothesis.

Is it ever necessary to intervene in this type of injury? The answer with a renal contusion is no, except in the one specific instance when there is an underlying pelvi-ureteric abnormality where clots may form in the renal pelvis and cause complete obstruction. In this situation, urgent drainage of the kidney may be necessary. Such a diagnosis may not become evident for 24 hours or more and it is most unusual for any action to be needed in the immediate period after the trauma. The prognosis from contusion of the kidney is excellent. There is rarely any long-term disability. One American series reported over 980 cases of renal contusion diagnosed on IVU without any long-term consequences (Cass and Cass 1983).

Renal Laceration

Lacerations are often associated with a penetrating injury in which the capsule is torn; there is extravasation of both blood and urine. This is always apparent on an IVU. In such lacerations, surgical intervention is rarely needed in the acute phase. If one does intervene in the acute stage, one ends up removing the kidney in about 20% of cases. If surgery is delayed then there is still probably the same 20% nephrectomy rate. A long-term problem is caliceal obstruction which may require partial nephrectomy.

Rupture of the Kidney

In these patients an operation is likely to be needed. The IVU may show gross disruption of the kidney with little functioning tissue apparent. The patient is usually desperately ill, often with other injuries, and will be in a state of peripheral circulatory failure. The diagnosis and the need for operation can be decided by discovering how much blood has been given and what is the state of the patient. If 40 ml/kg (half the blood volume) has been transfused and the patient's condition remains unstable, then surgery will always be necessary. Trauma centres dealing with this type of injury in USA work to this rule.

The outcome of these patients with an isolated renal injury is excellent and no patient should die from a lacerated kidney alone. However, 94% of patients with a ruptured kidney will lose the kidney at the time of operation. One obvious problem is when the IVU has shown a solitary kidney. In this situation, every effort must be made to preserve the injured kidney, although this is not always possible.

Pedicle Injury

One third of these patients do not have a haematuria, do not have an expanding mass and are not unduly ill. Under these circumstances, it is often difficult to appreciate that the patient has a severe renal injury. If the kidney has been avulsed from its pedicle, it is not usually possible to organise an arteriogram to prove this and get the patient to the operating theatre within one hour. This duration of warm ischaemic time means it is more than likely that the patient will lose the kidney. In some experienced centres in the USA, acute intervention is practised in this situation and one-third of the involved kidneys are saved, but if, alternatively, the patient is treated conservatively similar recovery rates are seen. The overall impression from the American literature is that something in the region of 50% of all kidneys with pedicle injury can be saved. However, the nature of the injury is not clear in many of these studies. In patients that I have seen, in whom there has been complete disruption of the vein and artery, there has been no way that the kidney could have been repaired and saved.

Some of these injuries are actually severe *intimal* tears and are essentially internal arterial injuries, in some of which an attempt can be made to treat by balloon dilatation. There may be a situation where a patient comes in with acute tenderness or swelling in the loin and no haematuria, but a pedicle injury is suspected. An IVU shows no excretion on that side. An arteriogram is then performed to confirm the injury by which time, perhaps, 1–2 hours have gone by. The angiographic study may then show that only a trickle of blood goes through into the kidney: if there is no flow of blood into the kidney then it is probably too late to do anything. If there is good flow the situation can be treated conservatively, whereas if there is a trickle of blood probably it will fall into the group that may well recover on its own if left alone.

In a case just like this reported by Robert Whitaker, a balloon catheter was put up, assuming an intimal tear. Good arterial supply was returned to the kidney on a short-term basis, but a week later the kidney was virtually non-functioning.

A DMSA scan takes some 3 hours, by which time any hope of saving a kidney with an acute pedicle injury will have passed: so in the acute phase of evaluation, there is no place for such scanning.

Probably, anomalous arterial supply to the kidney may account for the survival for some of these kidneys after a major pedicle injury. Anecdotally, there are reports of kidneys that have been deprived of their blood supply for two or more hours and have recovered substantially, so the situation may not be entirely analogous with transplantation kidney survival.

The average time for an ambulance to reach a patient at the scene of an accident in the northwest of Great Britain is 20 minutes. A further half hour is needed to get the patient back to hospital and to commence treatment. One is therefore talking about a delay of at least 30 minutes in most patients before the doctor has seen and fully assessed the patient. If the time to operation is added, then it must be accepted that perhaps 2–3 hours have gone by before the kidney is revascularised.

Our experience is not very large. I have performed nephrectomies for 3 ruptured kidneys. In one patient the spleen had to be removed as well because it was shattered. In another a hemi-hepatectomy was needed because the liver was damaged and acutely bleeding. In the third, there was a head injury and the patient was deeply unconscious. Thus, it can be seen that many of these patients have other major injuries. In some of the larger series that have been reported there are up to three additional major injuries apparent in the patients. Both the cases that I have seen with renal laceration were caused by blunt trauma. One of them had major extravasation of urine and the other only minor extravasation. Both were treated conservatively, but in one of them one-third of his blood volume was transfused. He stopped bleeding and never reached a loss of 40 ml/kg. Neither of the patients had other injuries: there have been no long-term consequences to either of them.

In patients with renal contusion, clot colic can be a very real problem leading to severe pain that requires considerable analgesia. Splinting or percutaneous drainage procedures have not been carried out and these patients have settled spontaneously with no long-term consequences. In our series we saw 3 patients with pelvi-ureteric junction obstruction, 2 of them acute-on-chronic. The history was of minor trauma, but the kidneys became acutely obstructed. In both patients the kidney was drained temporarily by percutaneous nephrostomy and both had a pyeloplasty three weeks later. Three patients had vesico-ureteric reflux as the underlying abnormality. There were two patients with horseshoe kidneys, one with possible pelvi-ureteric obstruction and the other without any obvious abnormality. This series covers the last 6 years of our experience.

Prognosis

One important aspect of renal injury is the need for medico-legal reports at a later date, increasing numbers of which are being requested. The emphasis here is on the prognosis following such an injury. The decision can very often be based on the appearances of the initial IVU and a follow-up study at a later date. If the injury has been a renal contusion only, then one can give an excellent prognosis. Even if there has been some delay in function as shown on the initial IVU, provided that these changes have recovered on the 6-month IVU, one can give an excellent prognosis. Compensation will be limited to the stay in hospital and the need for two or more sets of X-rays, but not for the long-term effects of renal injury. In the case of a laceration of the kidney, if the laceration has healed on a subsequent IVU and the kidney appearance is normal 6 months later, the prognosis is good. As far as pedicle injuries are concerned I cannot give much information on the medico-legal side because I have no experience of such kidneys being left untreated and my reading of the literature does not enlighten me as to the long-term problems that are encountered in this situation. I imagine that a guarded prognosis would be indicated.

I have not had any experience with acute disruption of the pelvi-ureteric junction, but from discussions with those who have seen such patients it seems that the kidney itself appears normal, but there is vast extravasation of contrast medium around it. Clearly the best procedure is immediate exploration of the kidney and repair of the pelvi-ureteric region. The results of such intervention should be good.

I have only seen one bladder rupture which was intra-peritoneal and this was apparent on IVU. The bladder was closed over a suprapubic Malecot catheter and the patient did very well.

Urethral Injury

I have had no experience of complete rupture of the urethra in children but I have dealt with 3 children with partial rupture. I investigated each of these by careful ascending cystourethrography which showed the damage, but it was perfectly possible to catheterise the child; a silastic catheter was left in place for 3 weeks. There were no long-term effects in any of the children.

It should be emphasised that the disruption of the urethra is frequently at the bladder neck level and not in the prostato-membranous region, as it is in adults. The choice is between simple suprapubic drainage or some method of realignment of the urethra in the acute stage.

Philip Ransley, who has to deal with the long-term complications, states that he would operate in the acute stage to realign the urethra in a male child, because the disruption often is at the bladder neck and not in the membranous urethra. The tissues are not as vulnerable as they are in the adult for late stricturing, and immediate realignment is likely to be successful. If the injury is at the membranous level then the risk of a subsequent stricture is exceedingly high.

Urethral injuries from intermittent catheterisation in a child are rarely seen. However, injured urethras after prolonged indwelling catheterisation are not uncommon. The whole anterior urethra can slough from the pressure effect of a long-term catheter in a child.

Philip Ransley would put in a plea for the use of DMSA scan in renal injury. A partial pedicle injury could be usefully studied with a DMSA scan. There may be a large haematoma around the kidney, but the DMSA scan will show whether there is still some useful functioning tissue within it. On exploration it is very difficult to see what tissue is worth keeping but, in two cases that he has explored after DMSA scans, he certainly found the scans helped enormously in this respect.

There are problems associated with renal biopsy. For the last 10 years, although we have performed one or two biopsies a week, only one serious injury to the kidney has been seen, in the form of an arterio-venous fistula which ruptured after 14 days. The haematoma expanded rapidly and it must either have compressed the kidney directly or caused complete obstruction to the outflow of urine. The physicians treated it conservatively at that time and the kidney has subsequently disappeared, as manifest by imaging 6 months later.

An open biopsy may be performed if physicians consider it to be too difficult by a percutaneous route. The problem with an open biopsy is that often one does not take enough renal medulla, especially if a wedge is taken. One is perhaps hesitant to go too close to the hilum of the kidney. Instead of doing an open biopsy, it is probably best to do a really careful percutaneous biopsy with a tru-cut needle under ultrasound control.

The need to biopsy the medulla depends on the condition under investigation. In most glomerular diseases there is a reasonably sized kidney which can be biopsied percutaneously. If one is trying to clarify a rare or obscure medullary cystic disease, a piece of medulla is necessary to make the correct diagnosis.

All severely injured testicles should be explored and the tunica repaired. This leads to more rapid recovery and probably helps to save some testicular tissue. If one is exploring any damaged organ it should always be made very clear to the parents that there is a substantial risk that the organ itself may need to be removed, and this should be implied on the consent form. Failure to do this could lead to medico-legal problems later.

Some practical aspects of the child with a contused kidney should be considered. How long does one keep the child in hospital if he/she still has haematuria from the contused kidney? We may know from the IVU and DMSA scan that there is no major disruption to the kidney. Does one keep the child in hospital until there is no macroscopic bleeding or until there is none on urine testing? Is one really worried about a late rupture?

If it is only a contusion and one is sure about this, the child can go home even with some bleeding still apparent. It would depend very much on how the parents felt about looking after the child at home. However, if there are medico-legal implications to the case or if the parents look as though they simply will not cope with the situation at home then the child should be kept in hospital until there is no evidence of macroscopic bleeding. If the child is perfectly well at a week but there is still some evidence of microscopic haematuria the parents should be encouraged that perhaps it is time for the child to go home.

Scanning by computed tomography in acute trauma is uncommon, but experience from Shreveport in the USA indicates that, in 14 children, the information that was obtained was better than from any other modality, although there was a half-hour wait for the scan.

An IVU should be done as soon as possible and certainly within the first 24 hours. The examination can be delayed until the next day in a child with macroscopic haematuria after a relatively minor injury in whom the clinical condition is satisfactory.

It is usually said that the hurry with a pedicle injury is not so much getting the patient to theatre but getting the abdomen opened as soon as the patient is anaesthetised. Before the anaesthetic there is always some vasoconstriction which closes the artery on a temporary basis, but the very moment that the patient receives muscle relaxants, the bleeding may begin in earnest.

Reference

Cass AS, Cass BP (1983) Immediate surgical management of severe renal injuries in multiple-injured patients. Urology 21: 140–145

Further Reading

Malek, RS (1976) Genitourinary trauma. In: Kelalis PP, King LR (eds) Clinical pediatric urology, Chapter 28. Saunders, Philadelphia.

Chapter 9

Intersex

Robert H. Whitaker and Philip G. Ransley

Intersex is a complicated subject. When one hears a lecture by an expert in this field such as Sir David Innes Williams, the whole topic appears entirely clear for the duration of the lecture. As soon as one is faced with a practical problem, however, all the information seems confused and the immediate diagnosis is not apparent. Therefore, we have spent some time in the last few months putting together a small booklet on intersex and this provides the basis for this chapter. This is a practical guide so that when the urologist is faced with an intersex problem at the bedside he will be able to contribute to any discussion with the paediatric endocrinologist and come to a conclusion as to what is best for the child.

There are two important factors that need to be taken into consideration when discussing intersexual disorders. The first is the *Mullerian Inhibiting Factor (MIF)*. This substance is necessary to suppress the female structures, uterus, Fallopian tubes and upper vagina, and to allow a normal male to develop (Fig. 9.1). The second requirement for development of a normal male is an intact pathway that allows the normal production and effect of *testosterone* on androgen-sensitive cells (Fig. 9.2). This pathway allows a normal androgen-sensitive cell to function correctly. The hormones produced by the pituitary induce the testicle to produce testosterone. Testosterone then enters the cell and is converted by the enzyme 5-alpha-reductase to dihydrotesterone (DHT). DHT combines with a binding protein and this complex enters the nucleus and influences the cell accordingly.

There are three possible sites for blockage along this pathway. First, there is a testosterone production defect and the example given here is the *17-ketosteroid reductase deficiency:* there are others. If testosterone is not being produced satisfactorily then there is an excessive production of androgen precursors. The second main defect occurs when the testosterone enters the

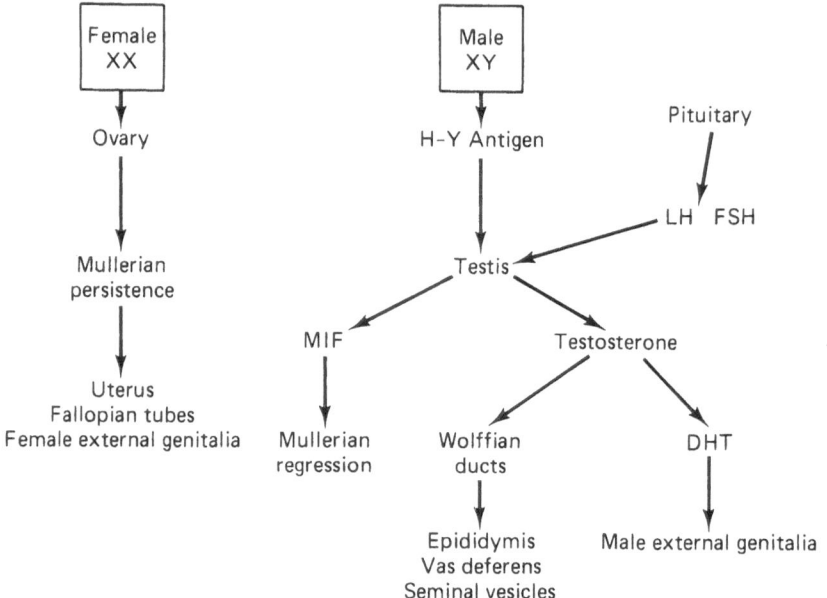

Fig. 9.1. The development of male and female structures and the influence of the Mullerian inhibiting factor.

cell; this is the *absence of 5-alpha reductase* to convert testosterone to DHT. The third defect is at the level of the binding proteins; if the binding proteins are abnormal, they will not combine with DHT, preventing DHT from acting satisfactorily on the nucleus. This produces the *androgen resistance syndrome* which can be partial or complete (previously known as the testicular feminisation syndrome). So, it can be seen that the "default value" in normal sexual development is female and that, unless there are proper pathways for the function of androgen sensitive cells and production of MIF, a female fetus develops.

Investigations

First of all, the physical examination must determine the size of the phallus by estimating the amount of corpus cavenosum present. Second, the site of the urethral meatus must be determined. Is the meatus on the end of the phallus or is it grossly hypospadiac? Third, is there a palpable gonad? If one can feel a gonad then it is almost certainly a testis. One must take the blood pressure, look for dysmorphic features and assess the degree of abnormal pigmentation. These features are all in reference to the diagnosis of *congenital adrenal hyperplasia (CAH)*. In the history one must determine whether the mother has taken any abnormal drugs, particularly oestrogens, during pregnancy.

Little emphasis can be placed on buccal smears as they are unreliable in the first two or three days of life. Chromosomes must be analysed for a karyotype

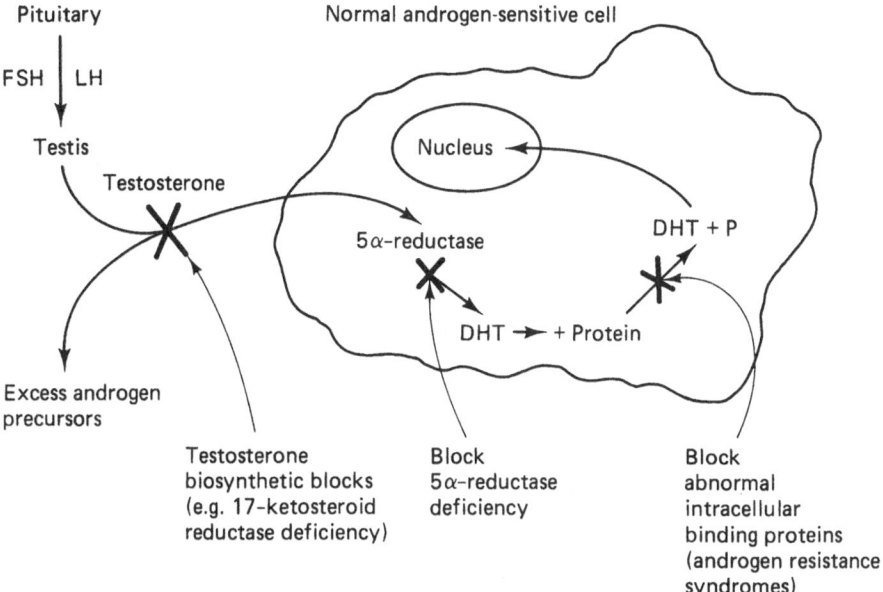

Fig. 9.2. The production and effect of testosterone.

and the biochemists in our hospital are able to give us a karyotype answer within 48 hours when there is an urgent need for a diagnosis in intersex. The plasma levels of 17-hydroxyprogesterone and 11-deoxycortisol are estimated. LH, FSH and testosterone levels should also be estimated. Cortisol and ACTH are useful, but not generally available. Urea and electrolyte levels are, of course, essential in reference to the diagnosis and management of CAH.

There are some other useful but not essential investigations in the early stages. These include an ultrasound to look at the internal organs, especially the uterus. This is particularly useful in the first few days of life when maternal oestrogens are still acting on the uterus, making it large enough to be seen on ultrasound. A genitogram can display the internal anatomy, but is not essential in the first few days of life. It is more useful later, when genital reconstruction is being considered. Diagnostic laparotomy was once quite popular but is rarely indicated now. It is still useful in a true hermaphrodite where biopsy of the gonad is essential for the diagnosis. We can now investigate androgen receptors by sending tissue to an appropriate laboratory to study the abnormal binding proteins.

Classification of Intersex

Intersex states can be classified into three distinct groups—*gonadal dysgenesis, male pseudohermaphrodites,* and *female pseudohermaphrodites* (Table 9.1).

Table 9.1. The classification of intersex

	Karyotype	Gonad	Genitalia	Clinical notes/treatment
Gonadal dysgenesis				
Turner's syndrome	45XO, or variant	Streaks	Female	Sexual infantilism, short stature, primary amenorrhoea, various inconstant physical features
Klinefelter's syndrome	XXY	Seminiferous tubule dysgenesis	Male	Small firm testes, aspermic, tall (long legs), gynaecomastia in 50%, may have mental and emotional difficulties
True hermaphroditism	46XX, 46XY, or mosaic	Ovary and testis, or ovotestis	Ambiguous or male	Variable internal and external organs, phallus, bifid scrotum, hypospadias. Surgery according to sex of rearing
Mixed gonadal dysgenesis	Mosaic (XO/XY)	Streak, undescended testes	Ambiguous or female	Short stature, mixed internal organs. Usually reared as female, but wide spectrum. Gonadectomy for cancer risk and virilisation
Pure gonadal dysgenesis	46XY	Streak	Female	Variable clitoral hypertrophy, failure of sexual development, primary amenorrhoea, gonadal cancer risk
	46XX	Streak	Female	No clitoral hypertrophy, no gonadal cancer risk
46XX Male	46XX	Testes	Male or ambiguous	Infertility, hypospadias, undescended testes, short stature. Genital surgery needed. Rare ++
Male pseudo-hermaphroditism				
Complete androgen resistance syndrome (Testicular feminisation)	46XY	Testes (undescended)	Female	Female external organs, short vagina, no uterus, breasts at puberty, gonad cancer risk. Due to defective end-organ response. Abnormal binding proteins
Incomplete androgen resistance syndrome (Incomplete testicular feminisation	46XY	Testes (undescended)	Ambiguous	Small phallus, variable labioscrotal fusion and virilisation, gynaecomastia. Due to defective end-organ response. Abnormal binding proteins

Table 9.1. *continued*

	Karyotype	Gonad	Genitalia	Clinical notes/treatment
Testosterone biosynthetic defects, e.g. 17-ketosteroid reductase deficiency	46XY	Testes (undescended)	Ambiguous	Male internal organs, severe hypospadias, short blind vagina, variable virilisation at puberty, variable breast development
5-alpha reductase deficiency	46XY	Testes	Ambiguous	Virilisation at puberty. Failure to convert T to DHT in androgen sensitive cells
Persistent Mullerian structures including – hernia uteri inguinale	46XY	Testes (undescended)	Male	Normal phallus, uterus and tubes (may be in inguinal hernia), poor sperm and hormone production, gonad cancer risk. Can be familial. Presumed failure of MIF production. Rare ++
Female pseudo-hermaphroditism				
Virilising congenital adrenal hyperplasia (e.g. 21-hydroxylase deficiency)	46XX	Ovaries	Ambiguous	Virilised, salt loss in 50%, uterus and upper vagina present, clitoral hypertrophy. Excess fetal androgen, raised plasma hydroxyprogesterone. Autosomal recessive. 1 : 10000 live births
Transplacental androgen	46XX	Ovaries	Ambiguous	Virilised. Exogenous androgen, or from virilising tumour in mother. Rare ++

Gonadal Dysgenesis

The gonadal dysgenetic group can be split into 6 subdivisions. The first is *Turner's syndrome,* which is 45XO, and its variants, in which there are streak gonads and the external genitalia appear female. *Klinefelter's syndrome,* XXY, is a true gonadal dysgenesis with tubular dysgenesis. These children are males. The third type includes the *true hermaphrodites* who are usually 46XX but there are areas, such as in South Africa, where they are more commonly 46XY. A true hermaphrodite has both ovarian and testicular tissue, but the gonad may be in the form of an ovotestis. The external genitalia are ambiguous. The fourth type is *mixed gonadal dysgenesis;* this is more common than most other types within the gonadal dysgenesis group. They have streak gonads and represent a spectrum of ambiguous genitalia, more often suitable for rearing as females, but some may be adequate males. The mosaic patterns that one sees in the karyotype are both different and distinguishable from the variations seen in Turner's syndrome. The fifth subdivision, the *pure gonadal dysgenetic* type, is excluded from this discussion as patients rarely present in the neonatal period. They are typically female patients with a streak gonad. The final subdivision is the exceedingly rare 46XX male. A careful study of the karyotype fails to show a Y chromosome. These children tend to present later with hypospadias and undescended testes.

Male Pseudohermaphrodites

The next main group comprises the male pseudohermaphrodites who all show the defects of testosterone production or effect on the androgen-sensitive cell. They are all 46XY. There are 5 subdivisions. The first two types are the *androgen resistance syndromes,* both complete and partial, that represent the problem of abnormal binding proteins within the cell. These were previously called the testicular feminisation syndrome. In the complete form of the androgen resistance syndrome, the appearances are female but there are testes present. The next type are the *testosterone biosynthetic defects* where there is ineffective production of testosterone from the testes. The example given in Table 9.1 is the 17-ketosteroid reductase deficiency. The children are 46XY with testes. Another defect, *5-alpha reductase deficiency* is seen most frequently in the Dominican Republic where children are born and brought up as females but then virilise at puberty; it has become an accepted phenomenon that they are then reared as males beyond that time. The reason for virilisation at puberty is the overwhelming production of androgens at that time, both from the testes and also indirectly from the adrenal. In the last type there is persistence of Mullerian structures as seen in the condition of *hernia uteri inguinale.* An apparent failure in production of MIF allows these male children to have persistent remnants of the female system in the form of a uterus and Fallopian tubes.

Female Pseudohermaphrodites

Female pseudohermaphrodites represent by far the largest main group in terms of occurrence. They are 46XX females. First, there is the type with virilising

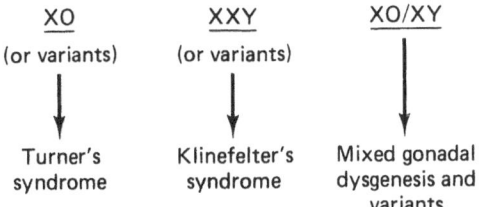

Fig. 9.3. Identification of dysgenetic group from karyotype.

adrenal hyperplasia, usually caused by 21-hydroxylase deficiency. Approximately 50% of these children have an obligatory salt loss. A second type, now rare, have virilised from the effect of transplacental androgen from the mother during pregnancy. This can be from exogenous androgen or from an androgen producing tumour in the mother.

Diagnosis

The diagnosis of these various conditions is best done by studying the karyotype. Fig. 9.3 shows how the dysgenetic group are identified simply from the karyotype. If there is 45XO or its variants then the diagnosis is Turner's syndrome. The XXY karyotype will diagnose Klinefelter's syndrome and the XO/XY gonadal dysgenesis group are similarly diagnosed.

If the karyotype is 46XX and the blood levels of 17-hydroxyprogesterone or 11-deoxycortisol are raised there is an instant diagnosis of congenital adrenal hyperplasia which can then be treated accordingly (Fig. 9.4). If the steroid profile is normal, the possibility of transplacental androgens must be considered: but this is now rarely seen. Another possible diagnosis to fit into this category of 46XX with normal biochemistry is the 46XX male, but he will be distinguishable by the fact that testes are present although they may not be immediately apparent. The true 46XX hermaphrodite could also fit into this group; such a diagnosis will be proved at laparotomy.

Finally, there is the 46XY group with ambiguous genitalia (Fig. 9.5). The resting testosterone levels may be of some value but they are not reliable enough to make a firm diagnosis. Therefore, an HCG stimulation test should be performed to detect the three different defects that have been described in the metabolic pathway of the androgen-sensitive cell. First, if there is a good response with excellent production of testosterone but no DHT, this must be *5-alpha-reductase deficiency*. If there is a good response with production of testosterone *and* DHT then there is an *androgen resistance* problem at the level of the binding proteins. Tissue should then be sent to a suitable laboratory for histochemical confirmation. Testosterone can be given to this group for 3 months. If there is no response in the appearance of the genitalia then the child should be brought up as a female. If there is sufficient increase in penile size for reconstruction, the child can be reared as male.

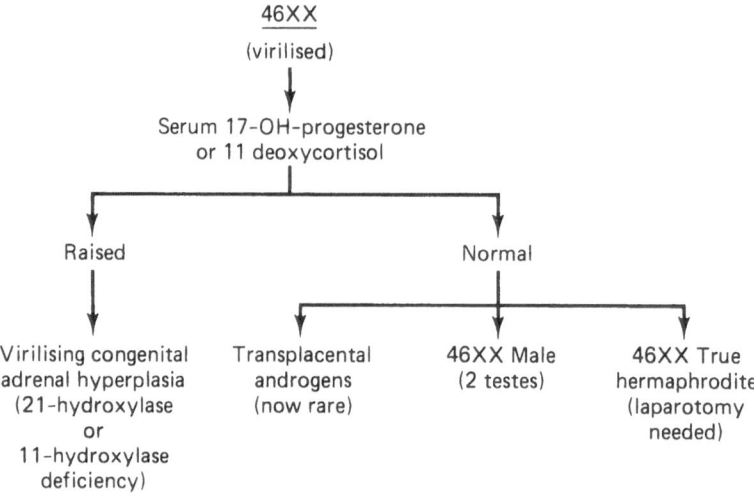

Fig. 9.4. Diagnostic diagram of 46XX virilised patient by biochemical analysis.

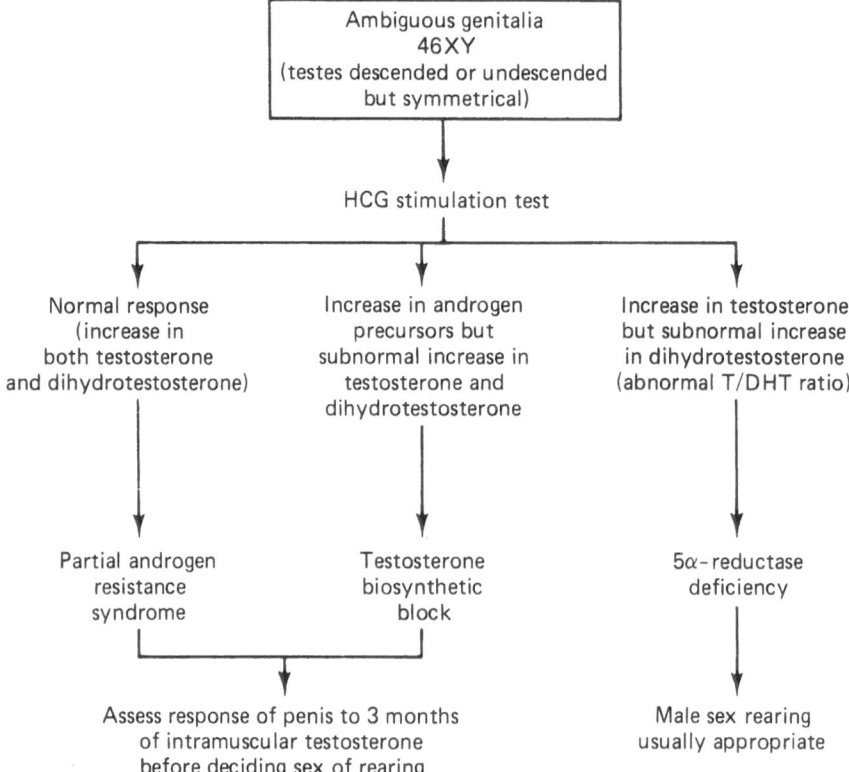

Fig. 9.5. Diagnostic diagram of 46XY patient with ambiguous genitalia, identified by the use of HCG stimulation test.

If there is low testosterone production with a high level of androgen precursors, then there must be a testosterone biosynthetic block such as 17-ketosteroid reductase deficiency. These patients should respond adequately to testosterone over a 3-month period. The penis should enlarge and the child can then be reared as a male, although a large amount of reconstructive surgery may be necessary.

Finally, other conditions may mimic intersex states and should be borne in mind. These include cloacal exstrophy, sinus abnormalities, micropenis and absence of the penis.

Special Problems in the Neonatal Period

Intersex must be put into perspective in the sense that 70% of patients with ambiguous genitalia who are seen by paediatric urologists will fall into the virilising congenital adrenal hyperplasia group. The diagnosis will be apparent within a day or two when the analyses come back for 17-hydroxyprogesterone levels; these results will probably be available before the chromosome analyses. The subject has been set out logically in this chapter and the situation should be clearly understandable. At the other end of the scale the complete androgen resistance syndrome will not be a problem in decision making. The problem cases in the neonatal period are the XO/XY mosaic, some of the true hermaphrodites and some of the XY male hermaphrodites. However, these only represent 10% of all the intersex problems. In this group of children decisions can be difficult, and often have to be made in association with endocrinologists.

One of the most difficult aspects is the ethnic problem. If a child has been pronounced to be male and it subsequently transpires that a female rearing would be more appropriate, the decision is often poorly accepted by parents in certain groups; this problem occurs especially in the Asian population. Because of ethnic difficulties, the children sometimes present late and parents will not accept any advice to change the sex of rearing.

The *XO/XY pattern* can represent quite a wide spectrum from what looks like a pure female through to grossly ambiguous genitalia with a large phallus that could be converted to an adequate penis. In the middle of this group there will be difficulty in deciding which way to go. Thus, if there is a moderate sized phallus with quite severe hypospadias, there are usually persistent Mullerian structures represented by the unilateral uterus and tube. There is a streak gonad on one side and a testis on the other, and one has to consider what surgery would be needed to put the situation right. If one decides on a male sex of rearing, laparotomy will be needed with excision of the vagina and excision of the uterus on one side together with the tube and the streak gonad. In addition there will be the need for an extensive hypospadias repair. To convert to female requires clitoral reduction and a feminising genitoplasty together with excision of the testis and the contralateral streak gonad. One must never leave a streak gonad in the presence of a Y chromosome because of the subsequent high risk of developing a gonadoblastoma or other tumour.

The final decision whether to rear as male or female depends primarily on the phenotypic sex and the response to testosterone. This applies in the XO/XY group, the partial androgen resistance group and the XY male pseudohermaphrodite group. In the end all is determined on the size of the phallus and its ability to respond to androgen stimulation. Therefore, one might need to undertake a trial of long-acting testosterone, 25 mg intramuscularly monthly for 3 months and monthly inspection of the phallus to assess growth. It is, however, only in the "grey areas" of these conditions that one needs to have a trial of testosterone. These are, inevitably, the most difficult groups to manage, particularly if, in addition, there are ethnic problems as there is a risk of being forced by the parents into making an inappropriate sex assignment.

Most of the patients with mixed gonadal dysgenesis are probably reared as female. There definitely is, however, a male end to that spectrum and rearing as male can be very successful. Surgical conversion to female is, of course, easier and if one is in the grey area the tendency is to opt for the female sex.

In reference to the testis, the streak gonad should be removed early but it would be nice to let the male child virilise spontaneously from the contralateral testis. A large series of tumours arising in such patients has been reviewed and the opinion was that it was safe to leave the testis until puberty.

It is similar to the problem of leaving the testes in the androgen resistance syndrome because these girls do feminise better if the testes are left until puberty to allow them to undergo a normal pubertal feminisation. It is, however, a problem to remove the gonads post-pubertally in any person. The gonads from girls with androgen resistance syndrome are removed routinely but it is most unusual to take out a testis post-pubertally in a boy with gonadal dysgenesis. It would be difficult to convince a boy to have his single testis removed when it is a good sized testicle which has developed well. Thus, opinions at present are against removing the testes. Provided that it is in the scrotum and is available for self-examination it can be left in situ; tumours that may develop tend to be benign. Leaving testes in girls with androgen resistance syndrome until puberty is not satisfactory and one should try to persuade the paediatric endocrinologists to let them be removed at an earlier stage.

The psychological aspects are very important. If the children are unhappy then probably one has made the incorrect decision. The unhappiest patients are not those in the intersex states but the children with absent penis and those with micropenis. Characteristically, the androgen resistance syndrome girls are very happy and contented and the mixed gonadal dysgenesis group are also usually satisfied. There is probably little need to tell these children of their intersex states, but of course it will be necessary to tell someone that they will not be fertile. Children with an absent penis or idiopathic micropenis who are to be raised as females should have their testes removed within the first week of life. If one is making a sex assignment for some form of structural or mechanical anomaly such as cloacal exstrophy or congenital absence of the penis, the testosterone surge within the first 3 months of life has a lot to do with subsequent behaviour; in such patients the testes should be removed almost as a matter of urgency in the first week of life, and this is usual practice in the cloacal exstrophy and micropenis groups. The two most unhappy patients seen by the authors are examples of micropenis and absent penis who had their testes left in for the first year of life.

The XY pure gonadal dysgenesis group is a problem. The children should sometimes be reared as males; this condition shows a great spectrum from streak gonad, through dysgenetic testis to Sertoli-cell-only testes. A number of them will be very adequate males.

One must also consider the boys who are unambiguously male, but whose parents are concerned about the size of the penis. Adult urologists certainly see this problem. A paediatric endocrinologist should be consulted and the child examined. If the penis looks a little on the small side, the parents should be reassured that it is not grossly abnormal and this usually takes the heat out of the situation. However, the child should be investigated just to be on the safe side (see Chapter 12).

Further Reading

Dialogues in pediatric urology (1987) Gender assignment: a team approach. Vol.10, No. 5
Glassberg KI (1985) Management of intersex. In: Whitaker RH, Woodward JR (eds) Pediatric urology. Butterworths, London, pp. 67–86

Chapter 10

Hypospadias

David C. S. Gough and Philip G. Ransley

Introduction

The three components of hypospadias are a hooded foreskin, a ventrally sited meatus and chordee. The word chordee comes from the French word meaning a bowstring. The incidence of hypospadias is approximately one in 200 live male births, so that a region such as the one in which I work, with 50 000 live births per annum, would expect to see 250 cases of hypospadias each year. This allows plenty of opportunity for those with an interest in the condition to develop considerable skills in its treatment.

The embryology can be summarised as follows. The cloacal membrane breaks down in the perineum at about 7 weeks of gestation and genital folds begin to form on either side of that whilst the genital tubercle in front begins to enlarge. At 9 weeks, the meatal opening has closed as far as the base of the shaft of the penis and by 11 weeks closure reaches the end of the penis. The final formation of the meatus takes place as a result of a core of cells growing back in from the tip of the penis to join up with the terminal meatus. Thus, in brief, the cloacal membrane first breaks down; there are the genital folds which "zip" the penis up to the bottom of the glans; then a core of cells migrate in from the glans to give the distal urethra. Only when that is complete does the foreskin begin to grow over the end of the penis. This whole process is complete by the third month of intrauterine life.

The vast majority of cases of hypospadias are very straightforward and simple to deal with. Two out of every three cases of hypospadias have the meatus at the base of the glans with minimal chordee. It seems that this is just a failure of the terminal portion of the urethra to form correctly. Slight or

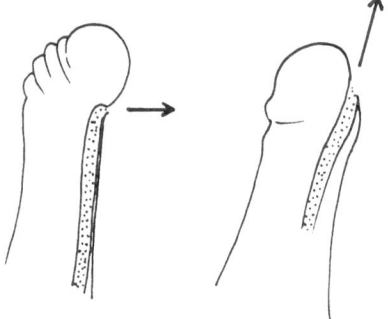

Fig. 10.1a, b. Deflection of the urinary stream in distal hypospadias by a bar of tissue beyond the meatus. **a.** Before a MAGPI repair. **b.** After a MAGPI repair.

moderate chordee occurs in about 25% of those with an opening on the distal shaft. The difficult cases of hypospadias that require 2–3 hours of surgery are, fortunately, quite rare representing 10% of all cases. The etiology of hypospadias is unknown but it was seen when oestrogens were given in early pregnancy; this is now a rare practice. There are chromosomal abnormalities in perhaps 5% of children with hypospadias and it is difficult to decide which should be investigated. Patients with a meatus at the base of the shaft need a micturating cystogram, to look for an enlarged utricle, and a chromosomal analysis. If severe cases of hypospadias are excluded then only 1% or 2% of cases have associated abnormalities of the upper tract, but they all have a higher than normal incidence of undescended testes. If one child in a family has hypospadias there is a one in 20 risk for further children being similarly affected.

Why do an operation? Even in children who have the meatus on the glans there may be difficulty in standing up and passing urine normally. There is a little bar distal to the meatus which deflects the urinary stream (Fig. 10.1). Some can compensate by angling the penis as they void, but occasionally this shuts off the stream as the urethra is compressed. The reasons for operating are listed in Table 10.1.

Table 10.1.   Indications for surgery in hypospadias

Practical	Awkward erections
	Voiding backwards or spraying
Psychological	Appearances

Pre-operative considerations

The decision to undertake repair of hypospadias is one to take individually. The incidence of hypospadias is high. It really is a common condition. Barry Belman quotes 8 per 1000 births, but of course the vast majority of these are distal hypospadias. The problem is that the repair of distal hypospadias is just

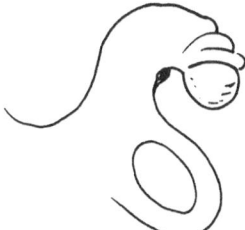

Fig. 10.2. Difficulty in classifying the meatus in hypospadias when there is severe chordee.

as difficult or more difficult than severe hypospadias. To obtain a good result in a minor condition without introducing any complications, but at the same time correcting those factors which you set out to correct, is a major challenge. One cannot decide to operate on only the simple types of hypospadias and not any of the more complicated ones. This is because the experience from both types is complementary.

The case illustrated in Fig. 10.2 shows the difficulty in classifying hypospadias. The more the chordee the more difficult it is to classify the meatus. This is because the coronal sulcus is at the peno-scrotal junction in cases of severe chordee. If testicles cannot be felt in a child with hypospadias, the alarm bells should ring. For instance, beware of a child with a testicle on one side with a vas and an abnormal epididymis and on the other side a tube, uterus and a small bit of vagina with a little streak gonad tucked away on the top. This is, of course, an XO/XY mosaic at the male end of the mixed gonadal dysgenesis spectrum and demonstrates that there are some XO/XY patients who can be successfully reared as males.

There are several questions to consider, when a child with hypospadias is examined.

1. Where is the meatus?
2. What difficulties does this create? The downward displacement of the stream is one of the primary indications for operation.
3. What is the shaft of the penis like? Is it small or is it of normal size?
4. Is there chordee?
5. What is the penile shaft skin like? Is it adequate to provide cover after the chordee is corrected?
6. What is the preputial skin like? Is there sufficient skin both to repair the urethra by whatever technique and to cover the shaft subsequently?
7. What is the glanular groove like and where is its position on the glans; this will also determine what technique can be used.

Fig. 10.3 illustrates a distal hypospadias with quite a deep glanular groove and plenty of preputial skin. The question is, has this child got chordee? His mother may be able to tell you what his erection looks like. Does this abnormality actually need correcting? The general trend is towards repair of minor degrees of hypospadias but if there is a problem it is often best to let the parents make the final decision. You explain to them that untreated the child will be normally fertile, and may be able to enjoy normal sexual activity but he will be left with two problems which are the risk of being teased at school and

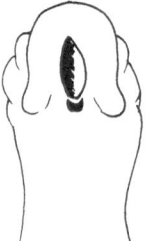

Fig. 10.3. Distal hypospadias with deep glanular groove and plentiful foreskin.

the abnormal direction of the urinary stream. Will he be able to pass urine satisfactorily through an open trouser fly with a parcel under each arm, having drunk three pints of beer? If he could cope with that then the operation is probably unnecessary. In a rather more severe case with a penile hypospadias, a nice deep glanular groove, limited ventral shaft skin and possibly some chordee but adequate preputial skin, it is usually quite clear that one could undertake corrective surgery as a single stage procedure.

The really severe cases with peno-scrotal hypospadias and an abnormal scrotum need further investigation. It is interesting to send tissue away from these children for androgen receptor studies since it is possible that there may be a degree of 5-alpha reductase or receptor deficiency and it may be that they will benefit from exogenous testosterone before reconstructive surgery is undertaken.

Even a child with peno-scrotal hypospadias but with two gonads in the scrotum should be investigated: one child (whose parents were both doctors) was not investigated although it was found later that he was a 46XX male. He was, therefore, treated with some testosterone before surgery, because of the small phallus, with some success. In summary, those that need investigation are the children with severe peno-scrotal hypospadias or any child with an undescended testis associated with hypospadias. The most likely diagnosis in a child with no palpable testes is congenital virilising adrenal hyperplasia.

Investigation of a 10-year-old Greek child with a well-formed phallus but no palpable testes showed that this child had non-salt-losing congenital adrenal hyperplasia. Although the paediatric urologist would have wished to keep this child as a male at this age, the parents insisted that the child should undergo surgery and be converted to a female.

Operative Considerations

Having decided to undertake surgery one needs to learn a spectrum of techniques in order to handle the various types of hypospadias (Fig. 10.4). Before undertaking the actual operation a decision must be made on timing. It is now accepted that the child is best operated on between the ages of 9 and 15 months, or between 3 and 4½ years. In fact 15 months is getting a little old and the limits should probably be changed to 7 to 13 months. With the use of foam

Chordee	Meatus	Procedure

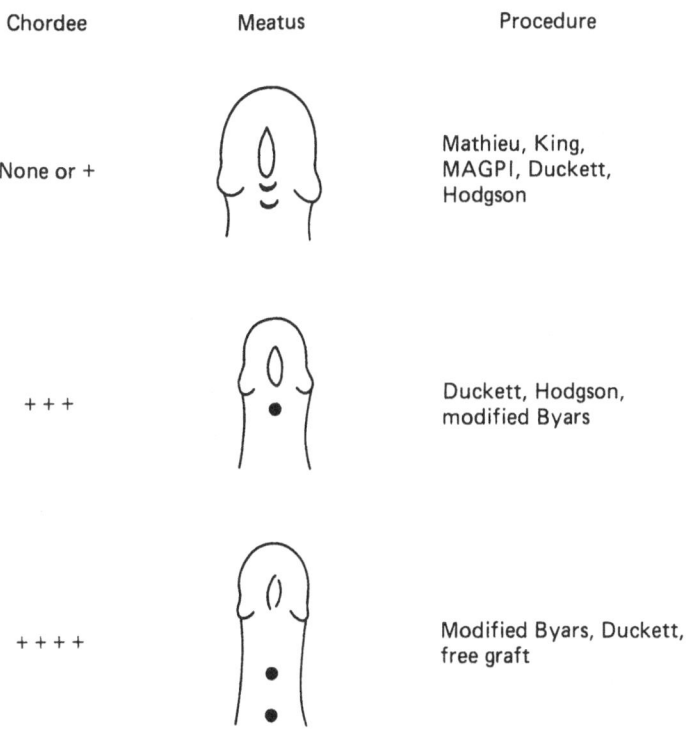

None or +		Mathieu, King, MAGPI, Duckett, Hodgson
+ + +		Duckett, Hodgson, modified Byars
+ + + +		Modified Byars, Duckett, free graft

Fig. 10.4.   Range and indications of operations for hypospadias repair.

dressings and 7/0 sutures it is a good time to perform surgery in these boys. If there are complicating factors then surgery can be left until later. The question arises of whether the child should have testosterone before hypospadias surgery; very few require it but it is something to be considered at least 3 months before the operation is due. Other associated abnormalities should be considered, such as constipation particularly in the group with ano-rectal problems. This is most important because one of the major adverse factors affecting the outcome of hypospadias surgery is the presence of constipation. Another factor that contributes to success is caudal anaesthesia which gives an excellent field in which to work. The children have no pain when they wake up and a much smoother post-operative course generally. The silastic foam dressing, too, has played a very major role in the success of hypospadias surgery. It is comfortable and gives a gentle compression of the penis to about 25 mm of mercury on the skin surface and keeps oedema under control. It probably preserves some skin that might otherwise be lost.

The system of catheter drainage must be selected carefully. A simple balloon catheter is easy to use, but is probably not ideal in many respects since there is urine around the balloon at the base of the bladder. If the child does get constipated in the post-operative period and starts straining, that urine gets forced out around the catheter. Furthermore, one has to pull the collapsed balloon through the repair 10 days after surgery and this is not ideal. A small silastic splint through the repair is more appropriate together with a suprapubic catheter; the "Duckett dripping splint", which is being used more often, may be better still. This is a simple silastic tube which runs right through into the bladder with a silastic dressing around the penis. The child wears a double nappy post-operatively: the inside nappy has a hole cut through it for the splint and the second nappy catches the drips of urine. The positioning of the splint is critical; if it is put too far into the bladder it will kink. It must be positioned in the bladder so that urine flows freely through it; it is then withdrawn until the urine flow stops. It is readvanced about 2 cm from this point and fixed with a prolene stitch through the glans.

A side hole in the catheter as well as an end hole gives a weak spot for the catheter to kink. The dripping stent may be quite a good idea. It is coming into regular use because it allows the patient to be sent home early and the parents are quite capable of looking after it.

In the post-operative period relief of pain is important but a caudal anaesthetic helps enormously with this. However, the use of a lot of paracetamol makes the children constipated; a laxative from early on in the post-operative period is important, especially in those with ano-rectal problems, to make sure that they have their bowels open and that they are not straining at stool. Antibiotic cover may be given with a single shot of intravenous gentamycin 2 mg/kg on the operating table. Prophylactic antibiotics in the post-operative period are not necessary as a rule. For the bladder mucosal grafts, gentamycin, metronidazole and ampicillin may be given as a single dose in the operating theatre; for a more complicated case they might be continued for 24 hours.

It is unnecessary to cut holes along the catheter in the region of the anastomosis even though a little pus may be found around the tube when a catheter is removed. Silastic foam dressings are usually removed after a week. The penis always looks satisfactory when the dressing first comes off, but of course then swells up after a further 24 hours. It takes several days to come back to a normal size.

Surgery for Hypospadias

The first thing is to assess the degree of chordee and the best way of doing this is with an artificial erection. This is central to the whole plan for surgery. There is no point in proceeding with a repair until the penis is straight. In some cases, even when the tissue has all been stripped from the ventral side of the penis, there is still an inherent bend on the corpora. This is probably quite common in patients with severe chordee. In a review some time ago it was found that 13% of patients undergoing hypospadias repair ended up having a Nesbitt procedure for straightening of the chordee. Looking back, standards were probably a little too rigorous at that time. To perform a Nesbitt procedure the neurovascular bundle must be lifted off the dorsal corpora. A longitudinal or elliptical incision is made in the tunica which is then sewn up transversely to get an entirely straight penis. An ellipse of tunica is excised and closure effected with absorbable sutures (PDS–polydioxanone). Non-absorbable sutures are unnecessary since the cut edges will heal well.

There are so many techniques available for the actual repair that one must limit oneself. Basically the *MAGPI* (meatal advancement and glanuloplasty) procedure, the *pedicled preputial tube* and the *bladder mucosal graft* as a free

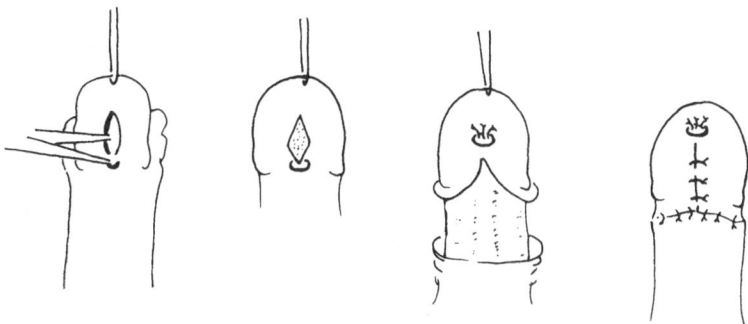

Fig. 10.5.   MAGPI hypospadias repair.

graft technique are used for the repair of hypospadias of increasing severity. The Mathieu repair in some hands gives rather poor results, though others get good results and it is increasing in popularity again. Magnification, 2½× or 3×, can be most helpful.

The *MAGPI* is a much talked about procedure; the principle is to alter the direction of the urinary stream from downwards or backwards to forwards (Fig. 10.1) and, incidentally, to improve the cosmetic appearance of the glans. The technique involves a vertical incision through the transverse bar which is deflecting the urinary stream (Fig. 10.5). It must divide this bar completely into the urethra. This incision is best done with a penile tourniquet and a fine sucker helps to keep the field entirely dry. The incision needs to be deep enough to recess the meatus well into the glans.

If there is a short dorsal reduplication of the urethra as there so often is in this situation, it can be simply divided with scissors so that the distal urethra becomes a single tube.

If the glanular groove is very deep, one does not need to cut as deeply with the incision. In fact, the best cosmetic results with the MAGPI procedure come from those with a deep glanular groove. The shallow glanular groove is a difficult one to get a good result from and may be best treated by a different technique such as the Mathieu or a free preputial graft. In principle the MAGPI operation consists of two Heineke–Mikulicz procedures. The first stage is division of the bar distal to the urethral opening; this area is closed by advancing the dorsal edge of the urethra to the far end of the incision (Fig. 10.5). The next part of the operation is a transverse incision just below the urethral orifice leaving 2–3 mm of skin. The incision is continued around the penis on the lines of a circumcision. The mid-point of this incision ventrally is lifted up and pulled forwards, and the transverse incision closed vertically pushing the tissue forwards to form a base of the urethra. The glans may need to be mobilised on either side just a little bit. There are many small variations on this theme, but it really can give an excellent result. Although it is only a relatively minor procedure it does correct the downward stream very effectively and gives a good cosmetic result.

An important point is that often one cannot decide on the exact nature of the operation until the patient is asleep and the area is inspected carefully. It is important to explain this point to the parents. The difference for the parents is the length of time the child is in the operating room, the type of dressing and the

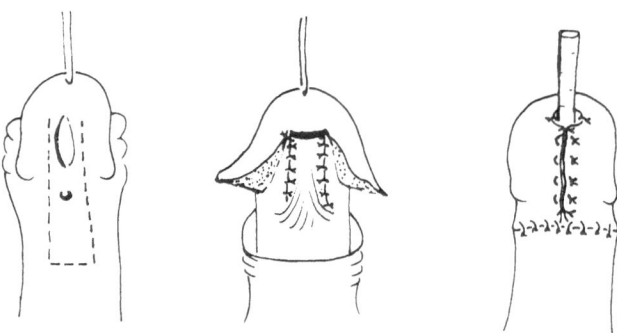

Fig. 10.6. Mathieu hypospadias repair.

duration of its application post-operatively. One should adhere to the principle that the incision in the skin must be proximal to the urethral opening to start with so that once the skin is all dropped back, it is possible to say whether the chordee has been adequately corrected; if so a MAGPI procedure can then be performed. Before cutting proximal to the meatus one must, of course, make sure that a Mathieu procedure is not needed. The Mathieu repair is a proximal based flap which is flipped forwards and has the glans rolled around it (Fig. 10.6). A variation on the meatal based flap is the Mustardé procedure in which the proximal meatal flap is rolled into a tube and then tunnelled through the glans. It is a good technique with an excellent cosmetic result but it is easy to get a stricture with this operation and it does require exceedingly delicate surgery. In general the Mathieu repair is applicable when there is a deep glanular groove whereas the Mustardé is more appropriate when there is a shallow glanular groove.

Two-stage repairs are rarely required today in paediatric urological practice. The only exception is with a very complex hypospadias where there is inadequate skin and a bladder mucosal graft is planned as a second stage but the tissues are not good enough to receive a free graft as a primary procedure. The *Denis Browne operation* is now completely outmoded and few paediatric urologists are likely to see such an operation these days; many of the old Denis Browne operations are now needing revision.

The *pedicled preputial tube* (Duckett or Asopa) operation is the standby for major hypospadias repairs (Fig. 10.7). It is ideal for penile and peno-scrotal hypospadias. It is based on an inner layer of preputial skin which is rolled into a tube and used to substitute the urethra with a terminal meatus created either by tunnelling or by splitting the glans and covering it with glanular tissue. There are many technical details of this operation which are important but will not be described here. The best suture material today is probably 6/0 PDS (poly-dioxanone) or 7/0 Dexon (polyglycolic acid) on the tube and 6/0 or 7/0 chromic catgut on the skin. This single stage repair is suitable for most hypospadias of some severity. It is possible to combine the preputial tube anteriorly with a Duplay tube posteriorly to give a complete urethral reconstruction. If there does not seem to be enough skin for coverage after the procedure then a bladder mucosal graft can be used to replace the urethra.

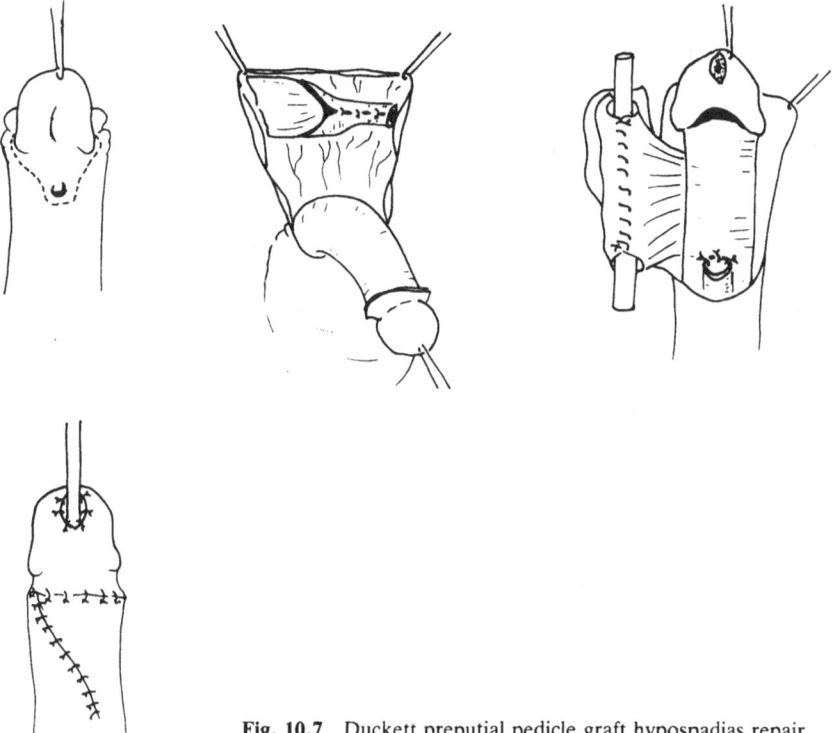

Fig. 10.7 Duckett preputial pedicle graft hypospadias repair.

The learning curve for this type of surgery is quite long as shown in Table 10.2. Each paediatric urologist must decide whether or not to undertake this type of difficult surgery; there is no doubt that hypospadias work will bring out all the weaknesses and increase the humility of even the best surgeon.

An alternative to the transverse preputial tube is an onlay graft in which the dorsal aspect of the skin is brought round as a double-faced flap. This is particularly useful for the longer penis where there is a strip-like defect on the ventral side. It is important that the skin is gently stretched before suturing otherwise too much skin is left and the result is a baggy appearance post-operatively. In order to excise skin without jeopardising the blood supply it is best to trim the penile skin and keep the foreskin.

Table 10.2. Learning curve for hypospadias repair

Year	Number	Fistula	Required dilatation	Partial skin necrosis
1979	12	9 (75%)	3	4
1980	16	4 (25%)	8	1
1981/2	32	3 (9%)	2	2

(13 (21% of total) required a Nesbitt operation for complete correction of chordee)

Finally the *bladder mucosal graft* must be mentioned. There is no doubt that this is an ideal technique and it is being used increasingly as a "rescue" operation. It does not seem to matter what tissue the free graft is laid upon and it seems unlikely that it does get any blood supply in the early stages from the corpora; it presumably gets its blood supply from the overlying skin. Postoperatively a suprapubic catheter is left in because the bladder has been opened to remove the mucosa. The repair can be stented with a silastic tube for 12 or so days. The tube needs to be somewhat bigger with a bladder mucosal graft and a 14FG splint could be used. Children who have a bladder mucosal graft seem to establish satisfactory voiding more quickly than children who have had preputial grafts. This is presumably because they do not acquire so much swelling. Strictures, of course, do occur with this type of free graft, probably due to a small area of the bladder mucosa not "taking". We have operated upon 47 patients who had had 140 previous operations. In total, we reconstructed 255 cm of neourethra; a mean of 5.5 cm per patient.

John Duckett has long experience of preputial grafts and his results are spectacular. He has a 4% fistula rate in 200 cases, which is quite remarkable. An interrupted suture is preferable to a continuous suture for the anastomosis and probably gives a water-tight closure. Careful stitching is essential. The pedicle may be wrapped over the anastomosis to try to get a bit more cover.

The proximal corpus spongiosum must be cut back until there is thick normal tissue; a thin piece of urethra must not be used for the anastomosis. The suture line must also be rotated round so that it lies against the corpora. Bleeding can be a nuisance from the glans, and adrenalin is used in three sites at the start of the procedure, at the peno-scrotal junction on each side of the urethra and in the mid-line of the glans itself. Bleeding is reduced if one leaves making the tunnel through the glans until after the tube itself has been constructed. Diathermy is rarely used on the penis during this operation.

Another important factor is that nowadays with the foam dressing there is no longer the worry at the end as to whether all the small bleeding points have been controlled. One final squeeze to remove any extraneous blood and then the foam dressing is applied, and when the foam is removed finally some days later the penis looks pristine.

Further Reading

Duckett JW (1985) Current hypospadias techniques. In: Whitaker RH, Woodward JR (eds) Pediatric urology. Butterworths, London, pp. 14–29
Whitaker RH (1988) Hypospadias: the MAGPI operation and fistula repair. In: Gingell C, Abrams P (eds) Controversies and innovations in urological surgery. Springer-Verlag, Heidelberg

Chapter 11

Neuropathic Bladder

David F. M. Thomas and Robert H. Whitaker

The neuropathic bladder is one of the most difficult but potentially rewarding areas in paediatric urology. Nowadays children with spina bifida have far less handicap than ever before because we are much more selective in those children who are treated; for many children, urinary incontinence is the only handicap. Among children with spina bifida 90%–100% have a neuropathic bladder. This has major implications for the children, for their education and for their families.

The normal methods of continence may be summarised. First, there must be a bladder of adequate functional capacity. This means that it must be large enough to allow the child to void intermittently every 3–4 hours. Second, the child needs voluntary control of the striated sphincter complex. Finally, there has to be volitional control of the voiding mechanism. In patients with neuropathic bladders, we are concerned not only with continence but with preservation of the upper urinary tract.

The normal mechanisms by which children gain continence are learned over the first 3 years. In the infant the pattern is of an unstable bladder with uninhibited detrusor activity. Young children void small amounts frequently, perhaps as often as 20 times a day at 1-year old. By the age of 3 years the functional capacity of the bladder is greater; the mean voided volume has increased about fourfold and the frequency of micturition is decreased to about 10 times per day. It is around this age that an element of volitional control starts appearing. This is a very complex pattern of learning and it is not surprising that things go wrong; a number of functional abnormalities can arise from derangement of this learning pattern.

History, Examination and Investigation

Children who have no obvious neurological disease, but who are wet, are referred to urologists. The most important point is to go into the history in detail. Are these children wet every single day of their life? Are they children who, for a period of weeks or months, have been dry? This is clearly of fundamental importance. Interestingly, many parents are keen to get their children dry at a very early age. Parents will say that they have had their children dry and out of nappies at the age of 12–18 months. This is somewhat spurious continence about which one should be wary, since some of these children will run into voiding problems later on. If the child has been dry for a significant period of time then it is very unlikely that one is dealing with a serious bladder neuropathy.

How wet is the child? Is there just a little dampness on the underclothes? Is it a patch of wetness that one can see through their outer clothes, or is it a puddle on the floor? Is it day-time wetting, is it confined to the night, or does it go on throughout day and night?

The child must next be examined carefully. The underclothes should be checked to see whether they really are wet since the parent's perception of wetness may vary very considerably from one parent to another. Is the bladder distended? It is most important to look at the spine. Are there any external stigmata of spinal dysraphism? It is important to check the knee, ankle and plantar reflexes and look at the external genitalia. Is there evidence of excoriation or an abnormality such as female epispadias? Is there any evidence of an ectopic ureteric opening? The examination is of utmost importance and nine times out of ten one has a very good idea what is going on simply from the history and the examination.

As far as investigations are concerned, an ultrasound is a very reasonable thing to do in any child with day-time wetting. As well as looking at the upper tracts it also shows the bladder before and after emptying. This gives quite a good idea of the post-void residual. An X-ray of the spine with appropriate views to show the lumbar spine and the sacrum adequately will indicate if there are minor degrees of sacral agenesis and spinal dysraphism.

Then there is the question of whether one should perform urodynamic studies. This inevitably depends on what is available and on the ability of the person doing the urodynamics. Urodynamic studies should be reserved for a selected group of children and not done routinely. There are, however, a number of studies on children with no obvious neurological disease, in which the pattern of bladder abnormalities is examined (Table 11.1). One of the things that varies most in these series is the percentage of normals. Top of the list of abnormalities is always detrusor instability. This condition is undoubtedly the most common cause of incontinence in children.

Table 11.1. Urodynamic findings in 60 children with non-neuropathic voiding disorders (Webster et al. 1984)

28 (47%)	Unstable
13 (22%)	Poor compliance
11 (18%)	Normal
5 (8%)	Large capacity bladder
3 (5%)	Small capacity bladder

"Non-neuropathic" Incontinence

Unstable Bladder

There is a group of children with the classic symptoms of frequency, urgency and incontinence who, on a post-void ultrasound, have no residual urine. However, there is also a group of children that are at some risk who have unstable bladders and have learnt to overcome the incontinence by excessive use of the external sphincter. This is a form of detrusor sphincter dyssynergia. These children have detrusor instability, but do not leak, and yet are generating high pressures; this is a potentially dangerous condition.

Treatment of the unstable bladder is primarily with anti-cholinergics and oxybutynin is the favoured drug at present, although imipramine and prob-anthine are useful as well. The learning of a voiding regimen is also most important. One does not understand the reasons for bladder instability because the whole mechanism of bladder control is so difficult to understand. However, getting children to empty their bladders at regular intervals is a vital part of the management even in children with an apparently small bladder capacity. In some of these children the symptoms are complicated by a urinary tract infection and they can be put onto prophylactic trimethoprim for a time. They are, however, a difficult group to treat, especially those with marked urgency and frequency. Some do not respond to anti-cholinergics and the only treat-ment one can offer at that time is reassurance that this is something from which many children suffer and that it is likely to improve in time.

The Low Pressure, High Capacity Bladder

The second group of problem children are those with low pressure, high capacity bladders. Again, this is almost certainly a functional abnormality and analogous with acquired megarectum. Indeed, it is not at all uncommon to find that these children also suffer from constipation. Something has gone wrong with the learning process, they do not empty their bladders and they get used to carrying around large volumes. They void incompletely and it is almost as though the mechanism has been reset so that they can disregard a sensation that would have other children hurrying off to the lavatory. Some of these children leak, others do not. Quite a few of them have urinary tract infections which should be treated rigorously. One has to explain to the parents that this is a condition which has developed over months or years, that it is not going to disappear overnight but that, with the co-operation of the parents and the child, it can be resolved over a period of months or years. Again a regular voiding regimen is needed and one can reinforce this by providing the child with a small alarm such as a cooking timer. It should be set to go off every 90 minutes following which the child goes to void. Phenoxybenzamine is reported as being a useful drug in this group but is not always successful. Antibiotic prophylaxis is most helpful when one is first starting to treat these children since the last thing one wants is a urinary tract infection to complicate the initiation of the therapy.

Treatment of constipation is vital. A lot of these children are not keen on high fibre diets so should be treated with a faecal softening agent (Dioctyl Syrup) or Senokot. One has to be prepared to spend considerable time with the children and their parents. These are the commoner forms of non-neuropathic incontinence. The more severe forms emerge with the occult neuropathic bladder.

Occult Neuropathic Bladder

The occult neuropathic bladder behaves like a neuropathic bladder, but there is no overt neurological disease. This is probably a mixed bunch as some children probably do have a form of neuropathy; with subtler forms of investigation one could probably pick out abnormalities of the reflex arc and abnormalities of innervation. Some of these abnormalities are undoubtedly acquired and represent the severe end of the spectrum of dysfunctional voiding. It is potentially a very serious condition. Most paediatric urologists have seen children who have gone into renal failure and need dialysis or transplantation as a result of this occult type of neuropathic bladder. Treatment is not simple but involves attention to associated constipation, voiding habits and the use of anticholinergics.

Nocturnal Enuresis

This is the most common cause of incontinence. One must explain to the patients that in a sense this is a normal phenomenon for a large number of children (Table 11.2). Reassurance is most important in the management of the condition; parents must be assured that many of the children's peers are also wet at night. The cause of nocturnal enuresis is still basically unknown. Of all active treatments, the pad and buzzer has the most consistently good results but, for it to work, the child has to be well motivated. It is, therefore, probably a waste of time trying to get a child dry at night until the age of 6 or 7 years. The child must be able to set the buzzer him/herself and to understand how the alarm system works. He/she must put the pad under the sheets and change the sheets when woken up at night wet. There are now some excellent small alarms that have a sensor within a pair of pants and the sheets often do not need changing. Having said that it is a successful form of treatment, it can, of course, fail if the child sleeps through the alarm. There may be other children in the room who are woken, but not the child in question. In this situation it is probably best to stop, wait for a while and then try again. The pad and buzzer treatment can be reinforced with oxybutynin or imipramine, but more often these drugs are useful when there is some day-time wetting as well.

Table 11.2. Nocturnal enuresis

Age (yr)	Incidence (%)
3	23
5	18
9	11
13	6
15	1–2

Neuropathic Bladder

Meningomyelocele is by far and away the most common cause of neuropathic bladder in children but, since we are seeing fewer children with spina bifida, other causes of neuropathic bladder are becoming relatively more important (e.g. spinal dysraphism, sacral agenesis, and children who have had extensive pelvic surgery or treatment for pelvic tumours). All urologists are familiar with the classical appearances of the neuropathic bladder and this may be associated with severe reflux.

The treatment of neuropathic bladder has two principal aims. One is to preserve renal function and the other is to attempt to impart continence. The standard treatment in the past, of course, was urinary diversion—the *ileal conduit*. There are very few paediatric urologists now performing ileal conduit diversions. This is because long-term follow-up of this type of diversion shows increasing numbers of complications; the upper tract deteriorates and there are stomal problems. *Clean intermittent catheterisation* now plays a very major role in the management of the neuropathic bladder. Clean intermittent catheterisation (CIC) was introduced by Lapides in the early 1970s (Lapides et al. 1972). Crooks and Enrile (1983) compare ileal diversion and clean intermittent catheterisation (Table 11.3). Amongst children who had normal upper tracts before diversion, 19 deteriorated and only 9 remained normal; in those who started off with abnormal upper tracts before the diversion, the majority deteriorated. With intermittent catheterisation, those that started off with normal upper tracts maintained their normality. It has to be said that there is some evidence that this is not always the case with clean intermittent catheterisation; in small children, deteriorating upper tracts are sometimes seen. Those with abnormal upper tracts remained stable on intermittent catheterisation: only 6 deteriorated. Thus, clean intermittent catheterisation does seem a better way of protecting the upper urinary tracts than external diversion.

Is it necessary to perform *urodynamic studies* before commencing a child with a neuropathic bladder on intermittent catheterisation? Between 50% and 70% of children can be managed successfully on intermittent catheterisation, but doubt exists as to whether all children need to be subjected to urodynamic studies before commencing the treatment. Some feel that such studies can be reserved for those in whom the initial treatment is not successful, but others feel that urodynamic studies should be performed on all children with a neuropathic bladder and that management is impossible without it. They believe that the studies should be performed with video visualisation of the

Table 11.3. Comparison of clean intermittent catheterisation and ileal conduit diversion (Crooks and Enrile 1983)

	Status before	Stable	Deteriorated
Ileal conduit	Normal	9	19
	Abnormal	2	18
Clean intermittent catheterisation	Normal	64	0
	Abnormal	30	6

urinary tract and that the two studies should not be done separately. By using urodynamic studies, three groups of children can be found.

Failure to Empty

There are children whose neuropathic bladder fails to empty, either because they have an acontractile bladder or because they have an inability to strain. The latter are children with high cord lesions who cannot generate a high intra-abdominal pressure. They often have, in addition, detrusor sphincter dyssynergia which results in a functional outflow obstruction. Children in this group are probably the easiest ones to treat provided they are not generating excessively high intravesical pressures. They retain urine in the bladder and are suitable candidates for intermittent catheterisation. If they have an element of bladder instability as well, they may need to be treated, in addition, with oxybutynin to ensure that the intermittent catheterisation is successful. Intermittent catheterisation is only practical if the children can retain sufficient urine to stay dry between 3-hourly catheterisations; this is really the minimum interval. If it needs to be done by a nurse every half hour, clearly this is not a practical proposition. In females, if CIC does not work, there is the option of an indwelling catheter. An indwelling catheter is not a practical proposition in a boy. In the last 2 years we have had two patients in whom a catheter caused the urethra to split right open. External sheaths are not a great success in small boys; a sheath is difficult to keep on and the penis gets rather soggy within it. In boys, increasing dilatation of the upper tract can be a real problem and it may be necessary to perform a sphincterotomy to allow the bladder to empty more satisfactorily. The cost of this procedure is often new or worsening incontinence. Thus, children in this group are effectively treated with intermittent catheterisation.

Storage Failure

A second group comprises children who have storage failure. Children with such bladders are unsuitable for intermittent catheterisation. The inability to store may be due to marked detrusor instability, reduced capacity, poor compliance, or sphincter weakness. Clearly it is important to identify which of these factors is the cause of their storage failure.

Poor Storage, Poor Emptying

Finally there is a large group of what can be termed "the intermediate bladder". These are bladders that neither store nor empty effectively. They have poor compliance, they fill up, perhaps to 70 or 80 ml, and often maintain rather a high pressure. After filling to such a volume they start to leak and rarely seem to have any organised detrusor contraction. In addition there may be some detrusor sphincter dyssynergia. This comprises a rather large group of children who are quite difficult to treat.

The first cause of *storage failure* is sphincter weakness. There have been a number of reports suggesting that *bladder neck suspension* can be effective here followed by intermittent catheterisation. Tony Rickwood has reported favourably on this procedure (Williams, Katz and Rickwood 1988). However, there must be a bladder of adequate capacity when one is dealing with isolated sphincter weakness. The other alternative in this group is an *artificial sphincter*. It must be appreciated, however, that even in a child who has an artificial sphincter inserted there is still the need for the bladder to empty satisfactorily and it is necessary to explain to the parents that it may be necessary to institute intermittent catheterisation as well. Thus one has to be sure that both the child and the parents are going to accept intermittent catheterisation as a possibility after insertion of an artificial sphincter. There is a group of children with storage failure because of a small capacity bladder of poor compliance. In this group, an artificial sphincter would be of no use since very high pressures would soon be generated and the upper tracts would be at risk. In some patients the reduced capacity may be a functional problem and anti-cholinergic drugs may help. However, in the majority of these patients, surgery will be needed to convert a non-compliant, low-capacity bladder into a larger low pressure storage bladder but even after this, intermittent catheterisation may be required.

Augmentation

The standard entero-cystoplasty would be with sigmoid or ileum and would be a simple detubularised augmentation or, nowadays, a clam ileo-cystoplasty. There are certain criteria that are needed before considering augmentation and urodynamic evaluation plays an important role. First one needs to calculate the desired bladder capacity. A formula helps with this—25 ml/year + 25 ml. Then one can look at the urodynamic studies and see whether such a storage capacity is possible or whether it is at the cost of too high an intravesical pressure. A reasonable maximum pressure would be 35 to 40 cm of water. If the children are unable to store urine at a reasonable pressure and start to leak before they reach their normal capacity, then this "leak pressure" needs to be estimated. If it is above 40 cm of water one can reasonably predict that they will do well with a detubularised augmentation because the evidence so far is that most of these detubularised segments store urine at pressures lower than 40 cm of water. So if the child is not leaking with an intravesical pressure above 40 cm of water and if, by augmenting, one can bring the intravesical pressure down below 40 cm of water, there is a reasonable chance that the intrinsic outflow resistance will be sufficient to keep the child dry if the bladder is augmented. Kramer et al. 1986 showed that tubularised segments generate high pressures, but that detubularised ones generally result in safer pressure zones. They showed that ileum does not differ urodynamically from right colon when segments are of similar shape. Thus, it probably does not matter what sort of bowel segment is used as long as it is detubularised. Having said this, there is some evidence that detubularised segments do not always store at pressures below 40 cm of water. There is great interest at the moment in the United States in the possibility of using stomach as a form of augmentation material (Adams et al. 1987). Although it sounds a little bizarre it does seem to be associated with far fewer metabolic problems than colon or ileum.

Artificial Sphincter

The only artificial sphincter worth considering is the AMS 800. In adults it may be reasonable to put it round the bulbar urethra but, in children, it really must go round the bladder neck. It is generally accepted that the minimum age for artificial sphincter implantation is about 10 years. In the series described by Bernard Churchill from Toronto, there was a 70% success rate without revision (Table 11.4). The rest required a number of revisions and 10% were failures even in this highly selected group. Artificial sphincters have a limited but important role to play and one has to consider very carefully which children are suitable for them.

Table 11.4. Artificial urinary sphincter in children (44 patients, mean age 11.4 yr: Churchill et al. 1986)

70% continent	No revision
10% continent	1 revision
10% continent	Several revisions
10% failure	
Revision rate 30%	
Success rate 90%	

Other alternatives are worth considering. The Philadelphia group are against the use of the artificial sphincter because they appreciate that mechanical failure is a possibility and that the children are going to need such mechanical devices for a very long time; they have looked for other alternatives using the child's own tissues. There are a number of different ways in which such alternatives can be effected. One of these is the *Mitrofanoff procedure* (Duckett and Snyder 1986), using the appendix as a non-refluxing catheteris-

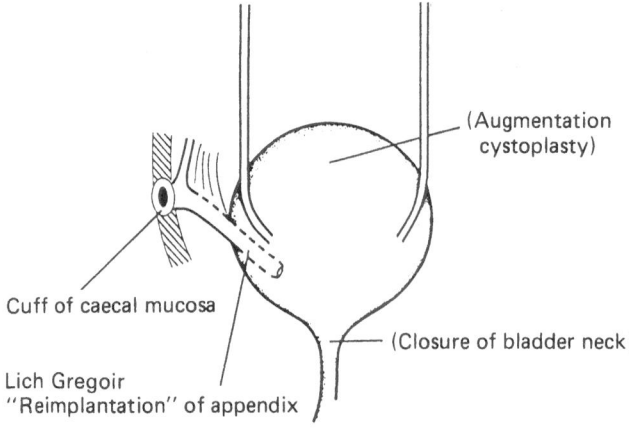

Fig. 11.1. Mitrofanoff procedure.

able stoma (Fig. 11.1), whilst one can also use the *Kock pouch* with a nipple or various other forms of drainage.

The urethral suspension operation consists essentially of a bladder suspension putting non-absorbable sutures on either side of the urethra along the lines of the Marshall–Marchetti procedure.

As far as the intermittent catheterisation is concerned, Ransley (personal communication) finds that a metal catheter is particularly good for girls. They are provided with 10 such catheters which are batch-sterilised in their tin foil so that the patients can go off to school with a couple of them in their school bag; this saves the need for washing the catheters immediately afterwards. Washing the catheters causes the girls most problems and embarrassment and appreciate not having to wash their catheters in a public place. There are metal catheters available with a mirror attached for teaching intermittent catheterisation. These are particularly useful. Self-lubricating 'LoFric' catheters are a significant advance in reducing discomfort, particularly for boys with some degree of urethral sensation.

References

Adams MC, Mitchell ME, Rink RC (1987) Gastrocystoplasty: a new solution to the problem of urologic reconstruction in the severely compromised patient. Data presented to Urology Section, American Academy of Pediatrics, 56th Annual Meeting, New Orleans

Churchill BM, Gilmour RF, Duffy PG (1986) Biologic response of the pediatric bladder rendered continent by artificial sphincter insertion. Data presented to Urology Section, American Academy of Pediatrics, 55th Annual Meeting, Washington

Crooks KK, Enrile BG (1983) Comparison of the ileal conduit and clean intermittent catheterisation for meningomyelocele. Pediatrics 72: 203–206

Duckett JW, Snyder HM (1986) Continent urinary diversion: variations on the Mitrofanoff principle. J Urol 136: 58–62

Kramer SA, Goldwasser B, Barrett DM, Webster GD (1986) Cystometric properties of ileum and right colon in patients after bladder augmentation or replacement. Data presented to Urology Section, American Academy of Pediatrics, 55th Annual Meeting, Washington

Lapides J, Dickno AC, Silber SJ, Lowe BS (1972) Clean intermittent self-catheterisation in the treatment of urinary tract disease. J Urol 107: 458–461

Webster GD, Koefoot RB, Sihelnik S (1984) Urodynamic abnormalities in neurologically normal children with micturition dysfunction. J Urol 132: 74–77

Williams MPL, Katz Z, Rickwood AMK (1988) Combined bladder augmentation and bladder neck suspension for neuropathic incontinence in girls. J Pediat Surg 23: 212–215

Further Reading

Bauer SB (1985) The management of spina bifida from birth onwards. In: Whitaker RH, Woodward JR (eds) Pediatric urology. Butterworths, London, pp. 87–112

Dialogues in pediatric urology (1988) Management of urinary incontinence in neurologic bladder. Vol.11, No.8

Chapter 12

Selected Topics

Robert H. Whitaker and Philip G. Ransley

Ectopic Ureterocele (see also Chap. 1)

Ectopic ureteroceles were discussed in Chapter 1, but more details may be given. There are two main ways of dealing with an ectopic ureterocele on the first occasion. A conservative operation can be performed where the upper pole of the kidney is removed with its ureter down as far as possible within the confines of a loin incision or a partial nephro-ureterectomy can be performed with a radical excision of the ureterocele and attention to the other ureters if necessary. There has been much debate as to which is the best approach and when each operation is indicated. In the short operation the lower part of the ureter is left open. It is not tied off but a drain is put down to it. On the next occasion that the bladder fills, the ureterocele will be squashed and its contents emptied upwards.

Although it is possible to perform a hemi-nephro-ureterectomy on the first occasion and simply wait to see how the child gets on most patients like to have the whole thing sorted out in one operation if at all possible. In the presence of severe infection, the procedure should be staged or, if possible, the urine should be drained for a while before any procedure is performed. If there is severe infection within the system, radiologists should be asked to put a percutaneous tube into the upper pole of the kidney. Only as a last resort should the ureterocele be cut endoscopically to allow the pus to escape because this then commits one to removing the ectopic ureterocele surgically in due course.

The rate at which one needs to go back to remove the lower ureterocele depends on the surgeon's threshold. The ureterocele has not been removed as a matter of principle since about 1980 in Ransley's unit and towards the end of this decade there should be some reasonable follow-up data. In George Kaplan's series or in the Boston series they were reoperating in well over 35% of patients. In the papers they stated that the patients required a second procedure. Whether "required" meant the surgeon decided that was what should be done, or whether the patients really did require a second procedure is difficult to know. There is no doubt that one of the worst forms of incontinence that one can encounter is post-ureterocelectomy. Examination of a lot of such patients who have had ureterocelectomy elsewhere reinforces the feeling that they should not have the ureterocele removed on the first occasion. This particularly applies to the caeco-ureterocele. Removal of this is a considerable undertaking since, by the time the ureterocele is excised, the urethra is open throughout its length right through the sphincter mechanism and a considerable amount of damage can be done removing such a ureterocele. The procedure is most difficult and the incontinence management afterwards is even more of a problem.

The MAGPI Operation for Hypospadias
(see also Chap. 10)

There are a few technical points that are worth discussing concerning the MAGPI operation. A very fine pair of scissors is used to cut the bar in the glans distal to the meatus. The cut is extended with the scissors to just short of the distal end of the glanular groove. It is a fairly deep cut performed whilst there is a tourniquet on the penis. The urethra is then held open whilst a suture takes a large bite of the posterior edge of the urethra, avoiding too much spongy tissue. This is then sutured to the distal end of the incision in the glanular groove. A mid-line stitch is used, and a stitch on either side, making three in all. Two stitches would probably be adequate. As John Duckett describes the operation, the next incision is just below the meatus and runs transversely across the ventral side of the penis. He then lifts up the mid point of the incision with a skin hook and sews the edges together below. This, however, can be done with a flat "V" incision with the tip of the "V" just below the meatus (Ozen and Whitaker 1987). This gives just as good a functional result and makes the operation considerably simpler. It means that the tissue that is approximated is less vascular because the incision does not extend into glanular tissue. At the edge of the "V" incision the incision is turned anteriorly again to begin the circumcision; this results in a "W"-shaped incision. The two points that make the bottom edges of the "W" are sewn together and this gives extended skin coverage below the meatus in the mid-line. This extra length of skin often means that it is then not necessary to transpose skin from the dorsal side of the penis. When one first starts doing the MAGPI operation one probably brings round the skin from the dorsal side too often and one is left with a baggy area of skin on the ventral side. With experience this is less likely to occur. The incision should be within perhaps 2 mm of the urethral opening so that, with closure of the skin, the meatus is advanced forwards even further. There is a danger of entering the urethra with the dissection because it is extremely thin at times. This can be avoided by making a deeper incision on either side of the urethra and then very carefully extending the dissection across the urethra at a somewhat lower level. It is then dissected forwards until there is a very small bridge of tissue, and once it is certain that there is no urethra within this bridge the tissue can be cut with a knife. When the ventral skin incision is closed it is only possible to put in three stitches. If a fourth one is attempted it often distorts the distal penis and this should be avoided. The need for visual magnification cannot be overemphasised; ×3 magnification is ideal but can be expensive.

The foam dressing deserves a further mention. Ransley pours the silastic liquid into the cover of a syringe, but others find that a polystyrene cup is most efficient (Whitaker and Dennis 1987). The cup is split so that the diameter of the dressing can be altered as the silastic is being poured into it. In this way it is possible to adjust the length and width of the dressing. It is important that the silastic solution is well aerated before use. The nurse who is preparing it starts stirring in air about 20 minutes before it is needed. The solution should probably be kept in the warm cupboard for half an hour before use as this allows it to set that much quicker once the catalyst is added. The silastic dressing, once it is set, needs to be fixed down and elastoplast is used around it which includes a little bit of the scrotum as that is the point at which it is most likely to ride up. It is essential to incorporate a 1-inch (2.5 cm) length of cocktail stick into the dressing: it lies under the loop of the stitch through the end of the penis. Incorporation of this bit of stick within the dressing stops the penis being pulled downwards out of the dressing.

With extremely delicate technique and using magnification, it is possible to close the vast majority of *fistulae* using a Y–V advancement technique. First the fistula must be dissected. A catheter is placed in the urethra and all the mucosa that extends through the fistula is excised. Any other mucosa drops back down within the urethral lumen. The tissues beyond the mucosa are then approximated with as many sutures as necessary, but avoiding the mucosa. It is sometimes possible to get a second layer of sutures in and then the flap of skin is laid across. There is no need for catheter drainage after this operation. Both the fistula and the skin are closed with 5/0 or 6/0 Vicryl (polyglactin).

The Diathermy Hook for Posterior Urethral Valves

Over the last few years, a hook (available from Cambmac Instruments Ltd, Pembroke Avenue, Waterbeach, Cambs CB5 9PY), has been used to destroy urethral valves (Whitaker and Sherwood 1986). The hook is made in such a way that it cannot catch normal tissue, but only something sticking out of the urethra, such as a valve. There is a very small area of bare metal within the hook that destroys the tissue when the current is applied. One of the advantages of the hook is that a general anaesthetic is not required and, because it is done in the X-ray department, one can see immediately by micturating cystography after the procedure that it has been successful.

The use of the hook has led, occasionally, to a little bit of bleeding or, on the odd occasion, to minimal extravasation, but nothing serious. One would probably see that after resection of the valve by any method. There have been no strictures yet. The diathermy current should be very low when using this hook. At the start, the diathermy should be on the very lowest setting and then turned up little by little until the job is obviously done. Once the hook is engaged it is often quite difficult to disengage it without first applying diathermy. Once the valve has been destroyed it is impossible to engage any tissue at all thereafter. The hook is designed as a disposable item because the diathermy current undoubtedly destroys the end of the hook eventually; once the insulation is no longer intact it should, of course, not be used again. The hook can be used as a diagnostic tool in boys with suspected pseudoprune conditions where there is a dilated urethra; the hook will determine whether or not a valve is present.

Duplication (see also Chap. 1)

Always think duplex! Consider the case of a young girl who would void normally, have post-micturition dribbling for 10 minutes, and then be perfectly dry for 4–5 hours. She has an ectopic ureter, probably passing through the sphincters. Although one often associates dribbling incontinence with duplex systems and ectopic ureters, the story is usually of continuous dribbling between voids. This case illustrates how difficult these problems can sometimes be. Always think of the possibility of a duplex system if there is a complicated case that you do not understand. Beware of strange appearances at the time of a micturating cystogram. Sometimes the catheter will enter an ectopic ureter at the bladder neck and demonstrate a large dilated system from the upper pole of the kidney.

Beware of the female child with a solitary kidney. Always think of the possibility of Mullerian abnormalities. These children present with periodic pain and normal menstruation at puberty; they distend one Mullerian system which is not patent and menstruate through the other patent system. Beware of the single ectopic ureter which can give incontinence in young girls. The kidney itself may be difficult to demonstrate as it is often poorly functioning but a DMSA scan can be useful. Although single ectopic ureters can give incontinence in females, they do not, as a rule, in males unless there is severe perineal hypospadias. Bilateral single ectopic ureters in females are very serious and a horrible problem. The kidneys are often dysplastic and the bladder is always extremely small. There is no development of the bladder neck and the child is incontinent. Even if the ureters are reimplanted these girls will continue to be incontinent due to the poor bladder neck development. The condition in females nearly always requires a bladder neck reconstruction, bladder augmentation and, probably, intermittent catheterisation. Many of them will later require dialysis and transplantation because they have dysplastic kidneys from the outset.

Micropenis (see also Chap. 9)

Unhappy people have already been discussed in Chapter 9 and perhaps the unhappiest is the boy with the micropenis; the penis is often no more than a piece of preputial skin. There are two types of micropenis. The first type is due to an endocrine problem whilst the second is a sporadic or dysgenetic micropenis. The majority of cases have an endocrine basis. Micropenis must be distinguished from a buried penis and, particularly, from a small buried penis.

A true *endocrine based micropenis* is a penis that is perfectly well formed with a meatus at the tip but which remains exquisitely small, below the normal size on the penile centile charts. The reason for this is either failure of the pituitary gonadotrophin mechanism (for example, microcephalics often have a micropenis), or it is a failure of the testes in terms of testosterone production. The penis develops in the first trimester of pregnancy under the influence of testosterone; its development depends on the conversion of testosterone by 5-alpha-reductase to DHT. Testosterone is produced from the testis by stimulation from chorionic gonadotrophin, and it is this chorionic gonadotrophin that is responsible for the development of the penis during the first trimester. In the second and third trimesters there is simply growth of the penis. During that time chorionic gonadotrophin becomes less important and the fetus's own pituitary gonadotrophin takes over. Therefore, with normal chorionic gonadotrophin there will be normal development, but failure of the infant's own pituitary hormone production or failure of the testes at a late stage to produce testosterone will lead to failure of growth and a micropenis will result.

Therefore, if one is dealing with a patient with a micropenis, the first thing is to establish the endocrine status by investigating the hypothalamic-pituitary-gonadal axis. This may involve performing an insulin stress test, an LHRH test and an HCG test to see if the axis is intact. Many of these boys will have a gonadotrophin deficiency such as that seen in Kallman's syndrome; the classical anosmia of this syndrome can be difficult to establish in a very small child. However, there may be a relative somewhere in the family who has similar gonadotrophin deficiency.

There are other gonadotrophin deficiency states that are not associated with anosmia. These children may respond to testosterone or HCG therapy by showing phallic growth. Although their penises never grow to anything like a normal size, they can be improved by giving testosterone early in life.

A *dysgenetic penis* is made of very poor material. The hypothalamic-pituitary-gonadal axis is intact. There is no endocrine treatment that is helpful and these boys will not respond to testosterone therapy. One may wish to consider gender reassignment in these patients. Some of these children are very unhappy and are best reared as females. This condition is particularly rare. Although it is not an intersex state, it is similar in that a diagnosis must be made early on so that appropriate treatment can be instituted. The psychological aspects of this situation are difficult to fathom, but the testosterone surge in the first three months of life is of enormous importance.

One must consider the child brought at about the age of 8 years by the parents who believe that his penis is not as large as it should be. One cannot be absolutely sure that this is not an intersex state and these children should be investigated endocrinologically. One has to exclude a slow-growing pituitary tumour. There is something in the concept of priming the tissue either in utero or early postnatal life so that the complete growth of the penis can be achieved at a later date. If the tissues are not primed then one never achieves full potential. At the end of the day it is the phenotype and the testosterone response that determines what should be done. One is certainly up against it when the boy is 8 years of age, particularly in certain ethnic groups. All those in the endocrine group should have a firm diagnosis made even though, in 99 cases out of 100, no other pathology is found on examinations such as CT scan; but there is a gonadotrophin deficiency in at least two-thirds of the cases. If they are gonadotrophin deficient, they should have a course of HCG to prime the testes and then a course of testosterone for 3 months to stimulate phallic growth. In most of these boys this produces reasonable phallic responses and they can be managed thereafter as gonadotrophic deficient children with replacement therapy at puberty.

If they do have an endocrine problem it is still possible that they may respond to treatment. It may be that there is a problem of timing in that they did not get the gonadotrophin surge in utero at the right time for the penis to be sensitised to subsequent stimulation. Such a child might respond to testosterone therapy. The dysgenetic group, of course, will not respond at all to testosterone.

Finally, one can summarise by saying that there are three groups of micropenis. A hypogonadotrophic group, a hypogonadal group and a dysgenetic group, but they are all quite rare.

The child who has a moderately well-formed penis but is clearly small for his age should be given a single dose of testosterone. If the testes are strongly retractile or slightly undescended then this is a good excuse to give some testosterone treatment and it can show the parents that the penis will grow adequately.

The Buried Penis

This is occasionally seen as a result of ritual circumcision with stenosis of the penile skin so that the penis becomes buried. The result is a similar appearance to the boy who has a true buried penis and has been circumcised; there is simply not enough skin to cover the penile shaft. The classical buried penis consists of preputial skin, scrotal skin and abdominal wall skin, but what is missing is what we would normally regard as penile shaft skin. The coronal sulcus appears to be at abdominal wall level. Many people would look at a buried penis and imagine that the phimosis of the prepuce is holding the penis in and that a circumcision would correct it. This is exactly what it fails to do. The operations that are designed to deal with a buried penis are most unsatisfactory. The corpora and penis are normally formed, but there is usually a fat pad around the penis. There is probably an abnormal attachment of the dartos muscle onto the penile shaft and coronal sulcus which holds the penis in. What can be done about it? Well, there is plenty of skin there that could be used to cover the penile shaft. The most appropriate operation for dealing with the buried penis is possibly to use the principle of the Duckett transverse preputial graft operation. The two layers of the prepuce are separated. The outer layer is used to clothe the base of the penis and the inner layer is separated into two segments which are wrapped round to provide skin cover for the distal penis. Anything less than this type of full mobilisation is doomed to failure.

There is no difference between a covered and a buried penis. They are both exactly the same. Operations have been devised for removing the fat pad around the base of the penis, but there is no useful purpose in this particular procedure.

There is no place for penile elongation operations in micropenis. They really do not work. If one looks at the geometry of the situation, it is hopeless. Freeing the penis from the bone will only rotate it downwards and backwards and this really does not help.

The natural history of the buried penis is a particularly important question because it is very tempting just to wait and see what happens to these children. With a good erection the penis would probably look entirely normal.

The indications for operation are that the boys are unhappy and are getting teased unmercifully at school.

The other condition to be discussed is *webbed penis*. There are older patients who genuinely do not like the way the scrotum is attached to the under surface of the penis and there is a case occasionally for dividing the scrotal skin and letting it drop back. The natural history of webbed penis is of interest. It may be seen in adults who have complained that they think it is unsightly and uncomfortable on erection, and it is possible to operate on both adults and children. There are two operations to deal with this. First of all one can do a very careful circumcision leaving plenty of skin on the ventral side which effectively lets the scrotal skin drop down. Alternatively, one can make an incision along the ventral side and let the scrotal skin drop back and leave the penis uncircumcised. A number of such children seen at birth in the obstetric hospital have been followed-up; some do genuinely improve spontaneously, but by no means all.

Megaureter

One of the difficult surgical problems associated with megaureter is the attempt to make the ureter narrow enough to fit comfortably into a new submucosal tunnel in the bladder. Anyone who has done a number of these operations will know the problems well and they will appreciate that the surgery is fraught with vascular problems in that however careful one is with the blood supply problems can arise. In theory the two factors that must be taken into account when a megaureter is narrowed are first that the operation of reimplantation is easier if the ureter is narrow, and second, and this is more in theory than in any practical aspect, that it is possible to regain active peristaltic activity in the lower ureter after it has been narrowed (Whitaker 1975). It is quite conceivable that when one has narrowed the lower end of a very wide ureter the top of the narrowed area may now represent, in effect, a pelvi-ureteric junction. In other words, this is the first point in the whole ureter where there is active coaptation of the ureter by peristaltic activity. This may be an important part of the reparative operation.

One operation in use now is the "keeling" operation that was described by Starr (Starr 1979). This is a more effective operation than the Kalicinski operation in which the ureter is folded (Kalicinski et al. 1977). It is most important that the top end of the keeled section should be funnel-shaped and not acutely narrowed. The technique is illustrated in Fig. 12.1 where it can be seen that the cross-section is similar to a horseshoe. Vicryl (polyglactin) suture material is usually used for this keeling procedure, but it probably does not matter very much what material is used. With optical magnification it is possible to pick and choose the position for the stitches in such a way that no large vessels are under-run. A psoas hitch is extremely useful to keep the submucosal tunnel long (Fig. 12.2). Without this there is a tendency for the bladder to contract down and for the tunnel to become much shorter post-operatively.

Post-operatively, on the IVU, one expects to see considerable resolution in an obstructed megaureter and a flat medial edge to the renal pelvis as it lies against the psoas muscle (Fig. 12.3). Coaptation is usually seen within the ureter and there may be a double shadow of contrast in the lower ureter after the keeling operation. Sometimes all the keeling can be done within the bladder, but usually it is more convenient to narrow the ureter outside the bladder. In order to do the psoas hitch satisfactorily the peritoneum needs to be stripped medially from its lateral attachments until the psoas muscle is exposed. Two large retractors and strong assistance are needed to expose the psoas muscle adequately.

The suturing of the lower ureter to the bladder mucosa requires a certain amount of ingenuity due to the rather strange shape of the ureteric lumen. However, this is usually not a great problem. If an excision tapering is being performed it is, once again, most important to make sure that the upper part of the tapered segment is funnelled, so that peristaltic activity can occur across this area. In either case the distal narrowed segment must be excised.

It is well worthwhile dissecting the ureter outside the bladder as well so that one can make sure that the ureter lies nicely before it is brought through the bladder wall to make the tunnel. The ureter can be brought about 1-inch (2.5 cm) down from the apex of the bladder with a psoas hitch so that if one did ever need to go back to readjust it there would still be plenty of bladder.

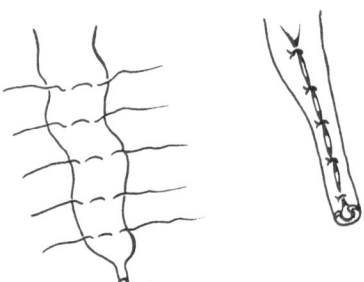

Fig. 12.1. Keeling of the ureter.

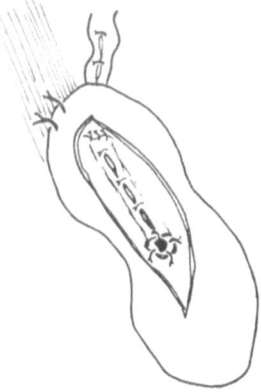

Fig. 12.2. Psoas hitch.

There is no place for simply incising the lower narrowed segment of a megaureter or treating it with balloon dilatation. This would be taking us back into the dark ages. This is the way that gynaecologists used to treat megaureters at the Johns Hopkins Hospital in the 1930s and 1940s. Many of these ureters were idiopathic megaureters and others were probably associated with tuberculosis. The etiology of megaureter is largely the inability of the wide ureter to form a bolus and hence there cannot be efficient transport of urine across the lower end of the ureter. This has been described in detail elsewhere (Whitaker 1975).

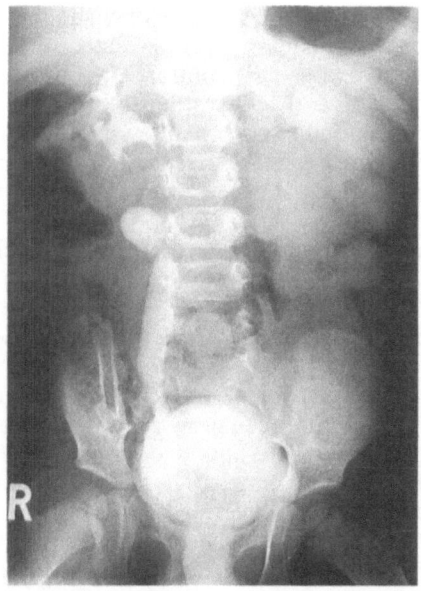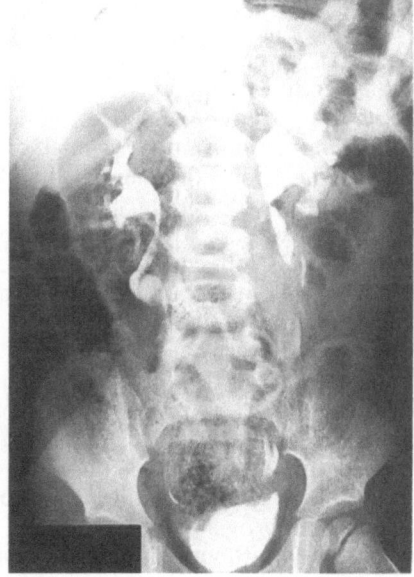

a   b

Fig. 12.3a,b. IVU before, **a**, and after, **b**, keeling and reimplanting of a megaureter.

   The Glenn–Anderson technique is of no advantage over the Cohen operation. In the Glenn–Anderson technique there is much less room for manoeuvre
and many of these abnormal ureters are already inserted well down towards the
bladder neck. Furthermore, the mucosa on the trigone is much more difficult to
lift than it is higher up. The theoretical advantage of Glenn–Anderson is that the
ureter lies in a physiological direction in the bladder, but it has been shown on
many occasions that taking the ureter across the bladder with the Cohen
technique is perfectly satisfactory. Another theoretical advantage of the
Glenn–Anderson is that a stone in the ureter at a later date would be easier to
remove endoscopically than after a Cohen operation.
   The basic principle of a reimplant operation for a wide ureter is a long tunnel.
The way in which the tunnel is kept long post-operatively, when the bladder
would normally contract down, is to perform a psoas hitch. The keeling is
simply to make the reimplantation easier and probably plays very little part in
the anti-reflux mechanism. If the ureter is not excessively large then, of course,
it should not be keeled. The alternative is to have a very long Cohen type of
reimplantation across the bladder, but this is inconvenient and rather bulky.
One factor that augurs badly for this particular operation is a lack of peristaltic
activity within the ureter as seen on fluoroscopy during a urogram. This is seen
in the non-obstructed ureters of the pseudoprune state and in the prune belly
syndrome itself. These ureters do not take kindly to narrowing which represents an increased resistance; to a particular patient this may result in
obstruction. It is advisable to avoid keeling or narrowing any ureter that does
not have good peristaltic activity. Perhaps one might be better to leave such a
non-obstructed aperistaltic ureter as an open hole into the bladder which could
reflux rather than to risk obstructing it.
   Conscious cystograms post-operatively in boys in whom the megaureter has
been reimplanted are performed at 6 months after the operation. If for some
reason a conscious cystogram is not possible, then a waking one should be
carried out. This is a particularly useful technique. After a cystoscopy, a
catheter is left in place, and the bladder is filled with contrast medium. A
manometer line is attached to the catheter and the anaesthetist is asked to
awaken the patient. As soon as the level in the manometer tube starts to rise,
bladder contraction can be assumed and the area is either screened or an X-ray
is taken. This is best done in small children. Older children seem to manage to
hang on and avoid voiding.
   It is not necessary to mobilise the bladder extensively before a psoas hitch.
Enough peritoneum should be removed from the dome of the bladder so that
the dome is freely extendable towards the psoas muscle without pulling the
peritoneum up with it. It is best not to disturb the opposite side of the bladder
or the other ureter.
   Some megaureters which seem obstructed appear less obstructed at a later
time because the whole of the lower end of the ureter can grow concomitantly
with the rest of the body. According to Pouseuille's law, a doubling of the
radius of the lumen will increase the flow rate 16 times. Therefore, a small
increase in the diameter will lead to a considerable lowering of the resistance
and clinical improvement. Having said that, very few megaureters do get better
spontaneously although admittedly many of them do not deteriorate over the
years.
   The etiology of the typical "rat-tail deformity" that is seen at the lower end

of the ureter which is often associated with a dilated spindle above it and slightly abnormal calices, could well be transient prenatal obstruction. Pressure studies on such ureters show no obstruction. If the condition is bilateral, the etiology may have been a transient prenatal bladder outflow obstruction.

References

Kalicinski ZH, Kansy J, Kotarbinska B, Joszt W (1977) Surgery for megaureter-modification of Hendren's operation. J Ped Surg 12: 183–188
Ozen HA, Whitaker RH (1987) Scope and limitations of the MAGPI hypospadias repair. Br J Urol 59: 81–83
Starr A (1979) A new concept in ureteral tailoring for megaureter. Invest Urol 17: 153–158
Whitaker RH (1975) Some observations and theories on the wide ureter and hydronephrosis. Br J Urol 47: 377–385
Whitaker RH, Dennis MJS (1987) Silastic foam dressing in hypospadias surgery. Ann R Coll Surg Engl 69: 59–60
Whitaker RH, Sherwood T (1986) An improved hook for destroying posterior urethral valves. J Urol 135: 531–532

Further Reading

Dialogues in pediatric urology (1985) Ureterocele management update. Vol. 8, No.2
Deane AM, Whitaker RH, Sherwood T (1988) Diathermy ablation of posterior urethral valves in neonates and infants. Br J Urol 62: 593–594
Whitaker RH (1985) Megaureter. In: Whitfield HN, Hendry WF (eds) Textbook of genitourinary surgery, Chapter 24. Churchill Livingstone, London

Subject Index